W9-AYF-229

CANNABIS OIL

QuickStart Guide

The Simplified Beginner's Guide to Cannabis Oil

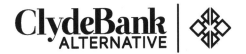

Copyright © 2016 by ClydeBank Media - All Rights Reserved.

This document is geared towards providing exact and reliable information in regards to the topic and issue covered. The publication is sold with the idea that the publisher is not required to render accounting, officially permitted, or otherwise, qualified services. If advice is necessary, legal or professional, a practiced individual in the profession should be ordered.

From a Declaration of Principles which was accepted and approved equally by a Committee of the American Bar Association and a Committee of Publishers and Associations. In no way is it legal to reproduce, duplicate, or transmit any part of this document in either electronic means or in printed format. Recording of this publication is strictly prohibited and any storage of this document is not allowed unless with written permission from the publisher.

The information provided herein is stated to be truthful and consistent, in that any liability, in terms of inattention or otherwise, by any usage or abuse of any policies, processes, or directions contained within is the solitary and utter responsibility of the recipient reader. Under no circumstances will any legal responsibility or blame be held against the publisher for any reparation, damages, or monetary loss due to the information herein, either directly or indirectly. Respective authors own all copyrights not held by the publisher. The information herein is offered for informational purposes solely, and is universal as so. The presentation of the information is without contract or any type of guarantee assurance.

Trademarks: All trademarks are the property of their respective owners. The trademarks that are used are without any consent, and the publication of the trademark is without permission or backing by the trademark owner. All trademarks and brands within this book are for clarifying purposes only and are owned by the owners themselves, not affiliated with this document.

Disclaimer: This publication is not designed to and does not provide medical advice, professional diagnosis, treatment, or services to you or to any other individual. This publication provides general information for educational purposes only. The information provided in this publication is not a substitute for medical or professional advice.

ClydeBank Media LLC is not associated with any organization, product or service discussed in this book. The publisher has made every effort to ensure that the information presented in this book was accurate at time of publication. All precautions have been taken in the preparation of this book. The publisher, author, editor and designer assume no responsibility for any loss, damage, or disruption caused by errors or omissions from this book, whether such errors or omissions result from negligence, accident, or any other cause.

Edition # 2 – Updated : June 24, 2016

Editor : Marilyn Burkley

Cover Illustration and Design: Katie Poorman, Copyright © 2016 by ClydeBank Media LLC
Interior Design: Katie Poorman, Copyright © 2016 by ClydeBank Media LLC

For information about bulk purchase discounts, please contact sales@clydebankmedia.com.

ClydeBank Media LLC
P.O Box 6561
Albany, NY 12206

Printed in the United States of America

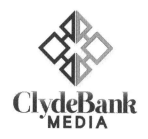

Copyright © 2016
www.clydebankmedia.com
All Rights Reserved

ISBN-13 : 978-1-945051-41-8

contents

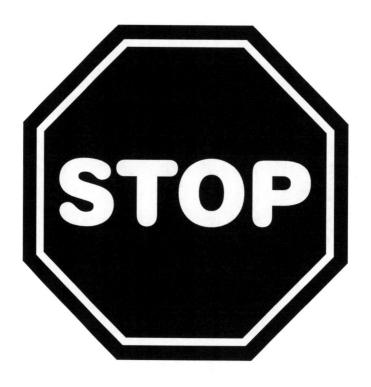

BEFORE YOU START READING, DOWNLOAD YOUR FREE DIGITAL ASSETS!

Be sure to visit the URL below on your computer or mobile device to access the free digital asset files that are included with your purchase of this book.

These digital assets will compliment the material in the book and are referenced throughout the text.

DOWNLOAD YOURS HERE:

www.clydebankmedia.com/cannabis-assets

introduction

When life and death hang in the balance, there's no time to make medical decisions based on politics. Many believe that prohibiting the use of cannabis, or marijuana, has disastrous implications, particularly the stifling of promising medical research involving cannabis oil. Regrettably, the production and consumption of this powerful medicinal tool is associated with hazardous in-home extraction processes, decades of recreational abuse, and violent black market exchanges. International transport of this medicine has led to severe and even capital punishment. Fire chiefs refer to the all-too-frequent in-home laboratory explosions and fires associated with cannabis oil as a societal hazard of epidemic proportions. In 2016, it was estimated that the decades-long criminality, as well as the legal, political, and social drama surrounding this plant, has tragically halted any thorough medical analysis of the product. We are left instead with sensational yet compelling anecdotal accounts of shrinking tumors and sudden miraculous relief from chronic inflammation and pain.

While prohibition-era-type politics and culture woefully stifled research on the medical front, it did generate a significant body of harm-related research. A consensus has thus emerged showing that the dangers of cannabis consumption are minimal when compared to those of many mainstream pharmaceuticals. Addiction potential is low and withdrawal symptoms are barely present. But after decades of poorly conceived law and narrowly focused, politically motivated research, asserting an objective vision on the topic of cannabis remains difficult.

Another factor that's left many unreceptive to the prospect of cannabis' potentially serious medical value is the fallout of the culture wars of the 1960s and 1970s. At such a polarizing time in the country's history, with the population divided along the lines of war and politics, the objective medicinal value of cannabis suffered immense collateral damage. In *Psychedelic Drugs Reconsidered*, a treatise on the overlooked medicinal value of psychedelics, Harvard professor Lester Grinspoon makes the case that the culture wars left a bad taste in the mouths of much of the establishment's medical community. Drugs like cannabis were grouped together alongside a whole litany of ultra-liberal political viewpoints and became in many ways "guilty by association." Grinspoon proceeds to extensively outline a multitude of clinical studies that have shown, if not conclusive proof, at least the promising potential of the value of psychedelics in traditional medicine. What makes Grinspoon's work particularly relevant is his ability to show in careful detail the growing disconnect between the dominant body politic and the objective findings of the medical community. It was this disconnect that set the stage for decades of propaganda and ignorance that would stunt medical advances while consuming the country in a costly and destructive drug war. It is our hope that publications like this one will gradually help to unravel fact from fiction and encourage a healthy, objective dialog on cannabis.

While the modern ignorance of potential curative, palliative, and analgesic applications for cannabis oil and other cannabis products is unwarranted and tragic, the political landscape appears to be softening. Nonetheless, corporate influence, particularly that of Big Pharma[1], will continue to pose a challenge to progress. Under the spell and fueled by the dollars of the pharmaceutical industry, doctors are often persuaded to discourage their patients from considering cannabis oil as an alternative

---

[1] The term "Big Pharma" refers to the pharmaceutical industry in general, but usually also the lobbyists that go to bat for these multibillion-dollar companies. The term has negative connotations that insinuate greed and a lack of compassion for the consumer.

treatment because "there's just too much we don't know." (Hence, another purpose of this book is to provide an exhaustive, levelheaded, and non-political account of what we at least *think* we know.) And while a growing brigade of green-rush up-and-comers are busy finding their fortunes in the cannabis medicine (and recreation) trade, the big players in the pharmaceutical scene would prefer that cannabis crawl back under the rock of misguided criminality from whence it came.

But what is it exactly that prevents major pharmaceutical companies like Merck and Pfizer from embracing cannabis and acknowledging and leveraging the plant's powerful medicinal properties to the fullest extent possible? In a word: money. In two words: money and patentability. The tried-and-true business model for any given pharmaceutical giant is Step 1) create in a lab, Step 2) patent in a legal office, and Step 3) set a steep price and enjoy a honeymoon period free from any generic competition. The outstanding medical potential of an organic drug like cannabis throws a wicked monkey wrench into this profit model. Not only is cannabis relatively inexpensive to produce, but—to the consternation of the pharmaceutical companies—cannabis is woefully difficult to patent. Its many strains, hybrids, and growing methods are a patent attorney's worst nightmare. Meanwhile, the thought of a cheap, non-patentable organic medicine—fueled on by a culture of activists, latter-day hippies, and common citizens who just don't want to be lied to anymore—competing with the laboratory-crafted Rx cash darlings is DEFCON 1 for Big Pharma. Worth noting especially are the multibillion-dollar cancer and pain-relief industries—two fronts where medical cannabis has serious market share potential.

Not to let the pro-cannabis side of this discussion off the hook too easily. The fog of war, disinformation, paucity of research, mistrust of government, etc., all created by the criminality of cannabis, has created a breeding ground for charlatans, unscrupulous green rush merchants, routine drug addicts, full-time quacks, and even moonlighting homeopathic physicians to make warrantless claims about the healing power of cannabis. Here's the problem with the political and intellectual texture of the modern counterculture: though less corrupt than the establishment, they're at times just as intellectually dishonest, either willfully so or by virtue of their ignorance and lack of curiosity.

It's a sociological problem, really. Having been confined to the shadows for multiple decades, cannabis producers and distributors and the proponents of cannabis medicine have had to operate at a disadvantage. When the substance in question is criminal to possess, there's no grant money available for research projects. There's limited capacity for centralized activity and academic peer-reviewed study. Meanwhile, the substance in question—cannabis—is ever dynamic and mercurial in its effects on individuals of varying physical, psychological and genetic makeup. Even the limited studies that have been conducted with cannabis are wanting for firm conclusions. The plant, seemingly by nature, has an ability to persistently avoid scientific consensus. Another interesting and complicating attribute of cannabis is the very personal and spiritual impression it leaves on those who consume it, either for recreation or medicine. Consumers of cannabis seem to have a unique and assertive confidence in their knowledge of the plant's physiological and psychological value. Such assertiveness, within a society that lacks much disciplined study on the subject, often manifests in claims (medical or otherwise) that are not adequately scrutinized. The nature of the cannabis experience bestows on the user a sense of authority and expertise, often forged by more abstract notions of spiritual experience and "journey." It also leads the user to erroneously conclude that the medicine's effects on him or her are indicative of its effects on others. As a result, the stark and often polar differences in the way cannabis consumption affects any given person (anxiety/relaxation, gregariousness/introversion, ebullience/grimness, hunger/inability to eat, etc.) is vastly underappreciated.

The political experiments being conducted in Colorado and Washington with the recreational legalization of cannabis have been by most accounts a resounding financial and social success—whopping revenue boosts for the state with no discernible uptick in costs. A time has come where other budget-crunched states and the Fed itself can't help but take careful note of what's possible via the reintegration of cannabis into the fabric of American medicine and sanctioned intoxication. While the green rush entrepreneurs flood into newly legalized states seeking new opportunities, large Canadian conglomerates such as Tweed take advantage of the country's newly minted "licensed producer" program, which allows a limited number of companies to produce and distribute massive quantities of cannabis and cannabis oil. South of the border, the agro-corporate behemoth Monsanto has won court cases reifying its ability to enforce patents on seeds, even hybridized seeds! Even when the consequence of such patenting makes entire crop yields unsaleable for small farmers. There's no doubt about it, Monsanto is ready to pounce should cannabis (and hemp) reassert itself as a legal crop. In anticipation of this move, a biotech company has begun to map the cannabis genome in an effort to make it more difficult for companies like Monsanto to pursue patents.

The purpose of this book is to provide a thoughtful accounting and review of what we know, what we think we know, and what we'd like to know at this unique moment in the political and medical history of this plant. Our main focus will be on the extraction and application of cannabis oil, which has garnered a significant amount of attention for its application in cancer treatment. This book will make every attempt to be objective and critical, seeking no political end, only a credible benchmark for where we currently stand with regard to leveraging cannabis oil as medicine.

| 1 |
A Brief Overview of Cannabis

What Is Cannabis?

The word "cannabis" is of Greek origin, likely derived from a Scythian or Thracian term. Three plant species make up the cannabis genus. They are *Cannabis sativa, Cannabis indica*, and *Cannabis ruderalis*, all originating in the Orient. Throughout time, these plants have provided tough fibers in the form of **hemp**, known for its broad industrial utility. Hemp can be used to produce items such as paper, fabric, biodiesel fuel, plastics, and nutritional supplements. The seeds, oil, leaves, and flowers of the cannabis plant are used as a medicine and a recreational drug. (Recently, compliance with the United Nations narcotics convention required the breeding of less potent hybrids containing less THC, the cannabinoid behind the complex physical and psychoactive effects on the human body.) The drug can be ingested in several forms, including smoking the female flowers and pressing or chemically extracting the flowers, leaves, and trim into extracts like hashish and oil.

The Anatomy of Cannabis

The cannabis plant is an annual flower. Its leaves are serrated with, at most, thirteen notched leaflets composing individual leaves. A unique arrangement of veins and leaf notches make distinguishing the plant from similar ones relatively easy. Absolute identification requires microscopic cell examination. The plants produce male and female flowers and are wind-pollinated. They are "short-day" growers, meaning that they flower when days grow shorter and nights are longer.

Cannabis plants manufacture cannabinoids, chemicals that affect the human body. The body creates cannabinoids on its own, which are known as endocannabinoids. There is some question as to the main function of the body's endocannabinoid system, but we know that it's a regulatory system that affects the way in which we remember, experience pain, experience hunger, and experience mood. The main mission of the endocannabinoid system is to keep us adequately balanced and stable. The binding sites for cannabinoids inside the body are known as CB1 and CB2, both of which were discovered in the early '90s and named after the cannabis plant, after it was found that cannabis produced its own cannabinoids (phytocannabinoids) that also bonded to these sites inside the body. Phytocannabinoids (commonly referred to as just "cannabinoids") are concentrated in the female flower parts. Dried flower buds are called "marijuana" and the resin, *hashish*. The drug is also available in extract or oil forms. Types of cannabis are grouped as follows: fibers, such as hemp, that are minimal intoxicants; high intoxicants; and related wild varieties.

The chemistry of cannabis is complex. Eighty-five cannabinoids affect the human brain, and 483 other chemicals are found in the plant. The chief source of psychoactivity is *tetrahydrocannabinol (THC)*, though another cannabinoid called *cannabidiol (CBD)* also plays a significant role in modulating the psychoactive effect by balancing out certain aspects of THC-related psychoactivity. Cannibidiol is a powerful neuroprotective ingredient with a tranquil, narcotic-like effect. For users prone to racing thoughts and anxiety from high doses of THC, using a strain with a proportionate quantity of cannabidiol to balance out the experience is a must. One of the nice things about using cannabis oil as the delivery medium for medicinal cannabis is that many manufacturers test and label their product for specific quantities of CBD.

It was cannabidiol that took center stage in the now-famous CNN documentary *Weed*, where Sanjay Gupta's investigation revealed how CBD's remarkable medicinal properties were put to use to drastically improve the life of young Charlotte Figi. Charlotte suffered from a form of epilepsy that was resistant to many traditional treatments. The frequency and severity of her seizures were dramatically reduced when she was given cannabis oil derived from a particular strain of high-CBD cannabis (which eventually came to be known as "Charlotte's Web"). The Charlotte's Web strain contained hardly any THC, so there were no psychoactive effects.

Creation of the high-CBD Charlotte's Web strain is credited to the Stanley brothers, a family-based Colorado growing operation that created Charlotte's Web by crossbreeding a strain of marijuana with hemp. They plan on expanding their production of this strain by moving their growing operation to Uruguay, where cannabis production and consumption are legal. They will then import Charlotte's Web into the United States as "hemp."

Other Noteworthy Cannabinoids

Cannabinol (CBN)

CBN can be created when cannabis is exposed to heat or air for a prolonged period of time, allowing the THC content to become oxidized. CBN is intensely sedative and can make you feel as if there's no reason in the universe to ever pry yourself away from the couch. As a medicine, CBN has certain antiemetic (anti-nausea) and anticonvulsive (anti-seizure) properties that are valuable.

Cannabigerol (CBG)

CBG is more prevalent in hemp, but growers have recently been keener on encouraging it in their cannabis plants as well. CBG

15

is a building block component of both THC and CBD. On its own, this cannabinoid produces certain antibacterial and tumor shrinking qualities that make it an asset to any medicine cabinet. When using cannabis oil to treat glaucoma, CBG is good to have on hand, as it reduces the level of intraocular pressure. CBG is also said to be effective at treating irritable bowel syndrome.

Cannabichromene (CBC)

Like CBD, CBC doesn't have a substantial psychoactive effect and is scarcely mentioned outside of medical circles. In truth, CBC is almost as prevalent in cannabis as THC. CBC promotes healthy tissue growth in the bones and brain cells while reducing the abnormal cell growth of tumors. CBC is also credited with pain relief and antibacterial and antifungal properties.

Working with Terpenes : The Entourage Effect

Cannabinoids, along with aromatic compounds known as *terpenes*, work together to produce a phenomenon known as the "entourage effect," whereby the various components of each cannabinoid and terpene produce a total effect greater than the sum of their parts. Terpenes can also be used to suit the preference of the consumer/patient. One of the major benefits of cannabis oil over other forms of cannabis is that, if it's prepared with care, oil can better keep intact the valuable terpenes and cannabinoids of the plant. Here is a list of terpenes that are commonly found in cannabis:

Pinene

The alpha- and beta-pinene terpenes are aptly named for their pine-like aromas. This terpene is associated with mental exhilaration and alertness. For consumers who have a predisposition to anxiety from cannabis, it's best to avoid pinenes. Cannabis oil heavy in pinene can be used to treat asthma, because pinene is a natural bronchodilator. Pinene. Just like pine-scented cleaners—is a natural antiseptic and can be used to combat bacterial infection. Oils with a lot of pinene are also a good remedy for medical cannabis oil users struggling with attention and memory retention. Some common strains of cannabis in which pinene regularly appears include Jack Herer, Chemdawg, Bubba Kush, Trainwreck, and Super Silver Haze.

Myrcene

This terpene is used as an antioxidant and anti-carcinogenic, meaning it's valuable to those looking to prevent or treat cancer. Since myrcene tends to induce relaxation, it can be useful for medical cannabis oil patients looking for an end to their insomnia or better sleep in general. Myrcene is also used to reduce inflammation and pain and to relax the muscles. Strains such as Pure Kush, El Niño, Himalayan Gold, Skunk #1, and White Widow are rich in myrcene.

Limonene

Limonene is characterized by a zesty lemon-like aroma. Cannabis and cannabis oil containing limonene are antifungal and antibacterial agents that will also ward off the damaging effects of carcinogens. Limonene is used to treat gastrointestinal disturbances, heartburn, and depression. In some studies, cannabis with limonene in its profile has been shown to destroy breast cancer cells. You can usually find limonene represented in the following strains: OG Kush, Super Lemon Haze, Jack the Ripper, and Lemon Skunk.

Beta-Caryophyllene

This terpene is a gastroprotective, good for warding off ulcers and other gastrointestinal disorders. Beta-caryophyllene also serves as an anti-inflammatory that can be used to treat arthritis and various autoimmune disorders. This terpene has the pepper-like quality and aroma that's responsible for the distinctive black pepper smell. In cannabis, it is most easily found in a strain called hash plant.

Linalool

The smooth lavender scent of linalool is used to treat anxiety, seizures, and depression as well as skin disorders such as acne and sunburn. You can find linalool in the following cannabis strains: G-13, Amnesia Haze, Lavender, and LA Confidential.

When selecting a strain of cannabis or a type of cannabis oil, you can customize your selection to your specific needs and preferences by reviewing the terpene profile associated with the product. Many dispensaries will make information about terpene content available to you. You can also use free online strain guide resources, such as Leafly (Leafly.com), to obtain info on various strains.

Classification Quarrels

Originally, the cannabis genus was classified *Cannabis sativa* in 1753 by Linnaeus, the Father of Classification. The French biologist Lamarck found a second species, *Cannabis indica*. Subsequently, other species were proposed, but not fully accepted. Twentieth-century investigation in the Soviet Union thoroughly muddied the taxonomy waters, so much so that the question of species became critical to those involved with drug offenses in the United States. Clearly, *Cannabis sativa* was a banned substance, so what defense attorney—while defending a client caught possessing or selling some other variety of cannabis—would not take the opportunity to suggest to the judge and jury that the substance seized in connection with his client's arrest was not, in fact, technically *Cannabis sativa* but some other variety? Biological experts were often called in by both sides, disagreeing and talking past one another—one of many visible symptoms of poorly conceived law.

In 1976, two scientists proposed two subspecies of cannabis, and others identified even more subspecies within the existing set. Research continues, but in the world of proper botany there are generally three types of cannabis thought to exist. Sativa, the most ubiquitous, is tall and loose and favors semitropical lowlands. Indica is a squatter plant that thrives in cool climates. Ruderalis is a catchall term for the wild plants of Europe and Asia. Reference to these types is often made in drug commerce when describing the proportional makeup of the product, e.g., "80% sativa, 20% indica."

fig. 1

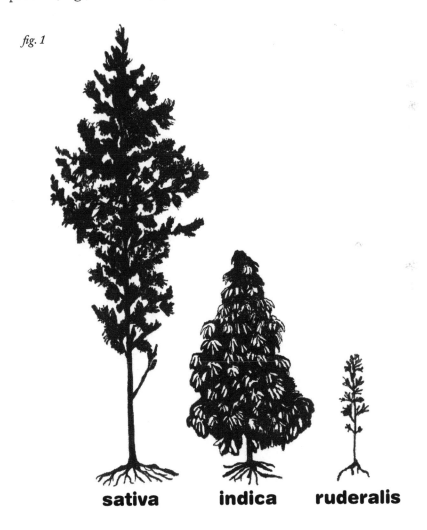

sativa　　**indica**　　**ruderalis**

Cannabis Uses

Hemp is the most common byproduct of cannabis. It is made from the plant's stems, which sometimes grow longer than eighteen feet. Versatile and strong, hemp is used in the paper and textile industries and serves as a construction material. It provides food in the form of milk, seeds, and oil. Evidence suggests that hemp has played a role in human industrial and agricultural affairs for the last 12,000 years.

The more sensational use of cannabis is, of course, as a recreational drug. Yearly usage exceeds 25 million people in America alone, while 100 million have reported that they've dabbled at least once. Its effects vary across individuals and include inducing a state of relaxation, giving a feeling of euphoria, and causing heightened introspection. In some cases, anxiety and paranoia are provoked. The appetite may spike and the pulse generally quickens slightly. Some cannabis users report the sensation of a racing heartbeat that is usually exacerbated by anxiety. There is also evidence that the risk of heart attack increases while one is intoxicated by cannabis. While this may be true, it should be noted that the risk of heart attack also increases (to the same extent or more) when you engage in vigorous exercise or sex. THC smooths out the arterial walls, causing an increase in blood flow (this is why the eyes redden after consuming cannabis) and a lowering of blood pressure. In some cases the heart rate responds by quickening its pace. This is normal and should not be feared. Unfortunately, people not used to experiencing the effects of cannabis can become alarmed by this uptick in cardiovascular tempo. The magnitude of these fears can be further increased by the effect of cannabis on the basolateral amygdala, the brain's fear-control center. The best approach to dealing with anxiety over an elevated heart rate is to 1) understand that it's a normal physiological reaction and 2) try not to dwell on your heart. Focus your attention on something else.

The effects of smoking cannabis typically fade in about three hours. Oral consumption invites longer effects, eight to twelve hours.

Cannabis sativa sparks energy and odd, excited behavior. *Cannabis indica* leaves the user "mellow" with its potent narcotic effect. Research suggests that the risks associated with cannabis use are lower than those associated with nicotine and alcohol. Excessive use may trigger short temper and sleeplessness. Withdrawal is not difficult.

fig. 2

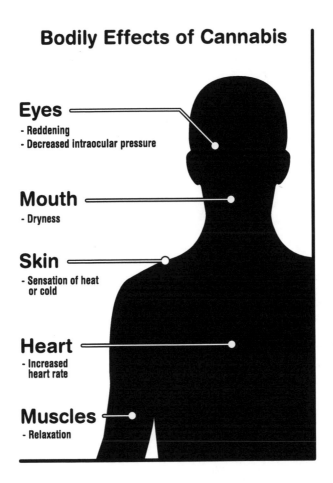

Bodily Effects of Cannabis

Eyes
- Reddening
- Decreased intraocular pressure

Mouth
- Dryness

Skin
- Sensation of heat or cold

Heart
- Increased heart rate

Muscles
- Relaxation

Earliest Times

Carl Sagan suggested that cannabis, and its botanical cousin hemp, were humanity's first agricultural products and the cornerstones of civilization. While that might seem a sizable claim, historical investigation definitely does trace cannabis back to China in 6000 BC. There, more than 3,000 years later, Emperor Shen Neng first used the plant for medicinal purposes. Over the next 1,200 years, cannabis use spread. Hindu India deemed it sacred and used it in rituals and as a medicine. Large-scale cultivation continued in China and spread to Scythia and Russia and on to Northern Europe. Cannabis leaves and seeds were found in a Berlin gravesite dated 500 BC. The Greek historian Herodotus recorded the use of the plant in rituals around 430 BC. In the Christian era, cannabis was stocked in the pharmacy of Nero's army and identified as a euphoric in the Talmud.

Around 3000 BC, hashish, which means "grass" in Arabic, appeared in Asia. It is the direct source of "hash"/cannabis oil. The *sadhus*, holy men of Northern India who devote their lives to asceticism and wandering the dimensions of consciousness, use hash in their ceremonies. The plant they use is locally known as *charas*, and it is thought to be descended from the same sacred plant used by the ancient Persians during their ceremonial "booz rooz." Hashish comes from the *Cannabis indica* that grows abundantly across the subcontinent.

Hashish is made by compressing and purifying any plant matter that contains *trichomes*, the tiny resinous glands that are most prevalent on the flowers of mature female plants. Hash can also be made using less trichome-rich portions of the plant, such as the leaves or trim. Mechanical separation processes include sieving or crushing to create powder that is then shaped into blocks with heat. The controversial practice of chemical separation is discussed in detail in Chapter 3. One point about that here: the extract is not technically "hash oil" because the trichomes are not in the liquid.

Over centuries, hashish and other cannabis products spread to the Middle East and then to Morocco. From there they reached other African countries. Around 1550, enslaved Angolans carried cannabis to Brazilian plantations.

The Dutchman Jan Huyghen van Linschoten provided the first Western documentation of cannabis. He described Egyptian and Turkish use, remarking on quantities eaten and the hallucinogenic results that followed.

Cannabis History in the United States

English settlers grew hemp in their Jamestown colony beginning in 1616. In the second half of the eighteenth century, medical cannabis joined other medicines in American and Scottish dispensaries. George Washington and Thomas Jefferson were both hemp growers. Plantations in the American southern states, as well as in New York and Nebraska, harvested untold amounts of hemp and cannabis. From 1850 to 1915, medical cannabis was commonly available at local pharmacies.

During the early twentieth century, the Mexican Revolution drove immigrants into the United States where their recreational, rather than medical, use of "marijuana," (slang for cannabis), soon caught on with the locals.

For the first ten thousand years or so of the plant's commercial, medical, and recreational history, governments largely maintained a laissez-faire attitude toward cannabis. That was to change in the United States when twentieth-century progressive-era zeal lumped cannabis together with alcohol and dubbed it an intoxicant.

The medicinal power of cannabis was disregarded in a rush to legislation, proponents note. In 1911, Massachusetts became the first of a series of states to ban it. While not specifically including cannabis, the Harrison Narcotics Tax Act of 1914 would lay the groundwork for its prohibition. It required all prescribers of opium or any of its derivatives to obtain a serial number from the Internal Revenue Department for each individual prescription. Every doctor who wished to prescribe narcotics was required to register annually with the federal government. Suddenly, there was a feasible infrastructure for government control over pharmaceutical distribution, an infrastructure that would mature and grow corrupt over the ensuing decades.

Elsewhere, in 1925, League of Nations members signed a treaty restricting cannabis to industrial and medicinal use only. It was red-flagged in the United Kingdom as a "dangerous drug" and, as such, prohibited.

In the 1930s, the Federal Bureau of Narcotics Commissioner Harry Anslinger, who claimed marijuana caused insanity and was a catalyst for criminality, and William Randolph Hearst, whose many newspapers pandered to these views, urged more restrictive federal legislation. They got their way with the 1937 "Marihuana Tax Act." While not a straightforward marijuana ban, the act's net effect was the same. Since the Harrison Narcotics Tax Act of 1914 didn't target marijuana, this legislation was the federal government's first true restrictive effort. The day the law was passed, October 2, 1937, two unfortunates, Samuel R. Caldwell, 58, an out-of-work laborer, and Moses Baca, 26, became the first marijuana seller and "possessor" convicted under US federal law. Caldwell did four years hard labor at Leavenworth and paid a one-thousand-dollar fine. Baca got eighteen months. Each man served his sentence in its entirety.

Ironically, these initiatives forced pharmacies to sell opium-based medicines like morphine as painkillers, to substitute for banned marijuana. Yet the reality of marijuana's medicinal benefits could not be completely thwarted. In the 1930s, major US drug companies Parke-Davis and Eli Lilly sold marijuana extracts as analgesics, antispasmodics, and sedatives. Grimault & Company marketed marijuana cigarettes as an asthma remedy.

In the late '30s, the forces of repression rolled on. Canada banned growing cannabis, and the United States dropped it from its pharmacopeia, destroying its reputation as a therapeutic. The **Boggs Act** of 1952 brought tougher sentences for sale or possession, two to five years. The subsequent Narcotics Control Act of 1956 upped the ante to two to ten.

Amid the storm of criminalization, there were tranquil seas of reason. For example, in 1938, New York City Mayor Fiorello La Guardia ordered the city's Academy of Medicine to study the effects of marijuana. The subsequent report concluded that many claims about its threats were unwarranted. Similarly, the 1968 Wootton Report, a product of the UK government's Advisory Committee on Drug Dependence, determined that moderate long-term cannabis use was not harmful. It concluded, "Cannabis is less dangerous than the opiates, amphetamines and barbiturates, and also less dangerous than alcohol."

The '60s era of sex, drugs, and rock and roll brought further federal bureaucratization, namely the April 8, 1968, creation of the Bureau of Narcotics and Dangerous Drugs (BNDD) by President Lyndon Johnson. As though to wish cannabis away completely, the ***Controlled Substances Act of 1970*** added that marijuana was "a drug with no acceptable medical use." President Richard Nixon, too, got into the act in 1971 when he announced on TV that, even though his White House Conference on Children and Youth voted to legalize marijuana, he felt "it would simply encourage more and more of our young people to start down the long, dismal road that leads to hard drugs and eventually self-destruction." Then he declared the first "War on Drugs": "America's public enemy number one in the United States is drug abuse," he opined.

This battle proved to be something of a Gettysburg for the anti-marijuana bloc. In the following years, consistent setbacks occurred. In 1972, the National Commission on Marijuana and Drug Abuse, also known as the Shafer Commission, recommended decriminalizing marijuana, and the National Organization for the Reform of Marijuana Laws petitioned the government to classify the drug to allow doctors to prescribe it under special conditions. The petition was granted— twenty-two years later! In 1976 the Netherlands legalized cannabis. In

1978 Robert Randall used the Common Law doctrine of necessity to defend himself against marijuana cultivation charges. He needed the drug for ophthalmologic problems. He won his case, and so became the first American officially permitted to use marijuana for medical reasons. That same year, the National Institute on Drug Abuse supplied seven individuals with *medical marijuana* via a "Compassionate Investigational New Drug (IND) program. It was also in 1978 that New Mexico passed a Therapeutic Research program which made medical cannabis available to a select group of cancer and glaucoma patients. New Mexico thus became the first of many states to legalize limited "Therapeutic Research" with controlled substances.

Marijuana matters took a sharp turn when, in 1980, the National Cancer Institute developed *Marinol*. This derivative of cannabis THC offered relief to seriously ill cancer patients. The government sold the patent to Unimed, and in 1985 the Food and Drug Administration granted the expected approval.

President Ronald Reagan took a step backward toward the bad old days when in 1986 he signed the Anti-Drug Abuse Act that imposed mandatory sentences for a variety of drug-connected crimes, exposing yet another shocking cannabis misconnect: owning 100 cannabis plants garnered the same sentence as possession of100 grams of cocaine. Later, matters were made worse when the act umpired a "three strikes and you're out" policy. This would mean life sentences for repeat offenders and death for "drug kingpins."

Offbeat religions, like Rastafarianism, had been using cannabis as communion. Elders of the Ethiopian Zion Coptic Church, founded in the United States in the mid-1970s, also imagined cannabis to be the Eucharist. A few newly founded Gnostic Christian sects see cannabis as the Tree of Life. Other cannabis-based religions sprang up like mushrooms after a heavy rain in the late twentieth century, for example the THC Ministry and the Cannabis Assembly.

The next twenty years marked the steady erosion of resistance to medical forms of marijuana, thanks to a jumble of court decisions, compassionate use disputes, opinion polls, drug rescheduling, marijuana laws, and studies. The air began to clear a bit when California became the first state to legalize the medical use of marijuana in 1996, followed in 1998 by Alaska, Oregon, and Washington. Other states followed suit over the next three years. Despite many states' legalization measures, the Supreme Court overrode them with its 2005 decision to ban medical use. The Food and Drug Administration (FDA) fell into line, stating that "no sound scientific studies supported medical use of marijuana for treatment in the United States, and no animal or human data supported the safety or efficacy of marijuana for general medical use."

But the tide of state legalization rolled on, reaching New York the day after Independence Day, 2014. The battle for medical use is not over, and the ensuing battle for recreational use has just begun. The general public has become more disillusioned with the decades of ignorance and fearmongering surrounding cannabis. CNN's Sanjay Gupta recently declared, "We have been terribly and systematically misled for seventy years in the United States."

Medical Cannabis

The term "medical marijuana" is used to describe an ostensibly limited use of the plant's THC and CBD to treat diseases and to relieve pain and disease symptoms. Though it's been a resource for physicians and other healers for thousands of years, cannabis use for mainstream medical purposes remains highly politicized and controversial, to say the least. Major medical organizations have spoken out against it. Its only widely accepted use thus far in the mainstream medical community is to control muscle spasms and to limit the nausea associated with chemotherapy treatments. Side effects seem benign and somewhat unclear. They include memory and cognition interruptions. Risks also exist concerning dependence and use by children and adolescents.

Relative to its pharmacological alternatives, cannabis often offers the most effective solution with the most minimal side effects. Cannabis has been used to successfully reduce pain caused by such diverse ailments as fibromyalgia and neuropathy, and is safer than painkillers composed of opium derivatives. A similar dynamic is maintained in the treatment of neurological disorders like epilepsy and multiple sclerosis, with cannabis providing a viable alternative to traditional treatments, and with no serious side effects. US agencies have given their blessing to Cesamet and Marinol, both used to reduce vomiting after traditional medicines prove inadequate. Other countries permit Sativex to combat neuropathic and cancer-caused pain. (Read more about cannabis use for specific diseases in Chapter 8.)

Nonetheless, the medical jury is still out concerning possible adverse effects of cannabis use. Experts point out mental and behavioral problems and liver disease connected with frequent indulgence. Evidence, albeit inconclusive, continues to mount suggesting that frequent and high-volume cannabis consumption can adversely affect neurodevelopment in teenagers and young adults. There are also studies that draw correlations between cannabis use and mental illness, though the causal link (proof that cannabis use causes mental illness) remains elusive. This is evidenced no better perhaps than by the lack of data supporting a causal link between cannabis consumption and schizophrenia. Though there is a well-documented *associative* link between cannabis use and a diagnosis of schizophrenia, the *causal* link has been all but historically disproven. While cannabis use skyrocketed in the 1960s and 1970s, the percentage of the population diagnosed with schizophrenia was unaffected, hovering at or near 1.5% of the total population.

fig. 3

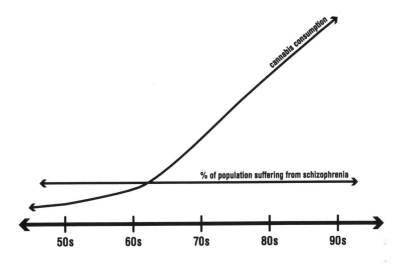

Cannabis Use & Schizophrenia

If cannabis use was indeed a culprit in producing a diagnosis of schizophrenia, then the '60s and '70s would have seen a noteworthy (and no doubt well publicized) uptick of diagnoses bestowed upon those "driven to madness" by this "dangerous" plant. Consider the undeniable causal link between tobacco smoking and lung cancer. As rates of tobacco use increase, so go the rates of lung cancer.

So what then are we to conclude about the fact that a greater proportion of schizophrenics, relative to the general population, consume cannabis? For one thing, we know that individuals with schizophrenia often seek relief from their symptoms through the consumption of cannabis. The "relief" obtained for the schizophrenic is thought to be temporary and, overall, cannabis consumption is thought to aggravate and accelerate the degenerative timeline of a schizophrenic. One longitudinal study (a study of several individuals over time) was able to document how people prone to schizophrenia, who were regular heavy cannabis consumers, were likely to be diagnosed with schizophrenia two to three years earlier than their non-cannabis-consuming counterparts.

The conclusion here is that cannabis, while it certainly does not cause schizophrenia in otherwise mentally healthy individuals, can accelerate the onset of mental illness in a predisposed individual.

Because the harm and risks associated with cannabis are limited, especially when compared to those of a multitude of other (mostly legal) drugs, the medical use of cannabis has escaped heavy censure. Many say it is safe. The US Food and Drug Administration and many physicians see the plant's cannabinoids as effective, but not when ingested in smoke and in quantities exceeding prescribed limits. They contend medical marijuana should pass the same rigorous tests as any new drug, a process that will take ten years or more. Cannabis oil presents patients with several ways to ingest smoke- and vapor-free baked goods (via tinctures) and cannabis-infused candies. Tinctures, in particular, can be ingested sublingually (under the tongue), which facilitates more direct absorption into the bloodstream compared to standard methods of ingestion. Eating cannabis-infused baked goods or candy produces a more enduring period of medical relief, though the medication must first pass through the liver, which can compromise the efficacy of CBD, one of the most medically potent cannabinoids.

Another important downside to oral ingestion is the relative difficulty of obtaining proper dosage. The effects of cannabis, when orally ingested, are delayed by thirty to sixty minutes, as opposed to smoking or vaping where the effects are immediate. Smoking or vaping thereby allow for better dosage control. For patients who are new to cannabis or who have an exceptionally low tolerance, vaporizing is the preferred ingestion method, because it allows the gentlest and most controlled absorption of cannabinoids into the body.

The story of "cannabis as medicine" is a dramatic one, filled with harrowing tales of heroes and villains and an ongoing search for truth, reason, and understanding. In the ensuing chapters of this book, we'll take a closer look at a few of the major dramas that have surrounded this most politically potent natural medicine.

| 2 |

Cannabis Oil Basics

Note : Before proceeding with the production or utilization of cannabis oil, it's important to understand the legal distinctions that exist between cannabis and cannabis concentrates. Even in parts of the country or world with more relaxed cannabis laws, there are often separate provisions regulating the production, sale, and consumption of cannabis concentrates. In weed-friendly California, for example, there's a statute on the books dealing directly with "chemical extractions" of cannabis:

> *Section 11379.6(a) states: "Except as otherwise provided by law, every person who compounds, converts, produces, derives, processes, or prepares, either directly or indirectly by chemical extraction or independently by means of chemical synthesis, any controlled substance – shall be punished by imprisonment in the state prison for three, five, or seven years and by a fine up to $50,000."*

Another law is pending in California that restricts a physician's ability to recommend certain types of cannabis concentrates to a patient. If this law passes it could radically alter the typical California dispensary's inventory lineup, since about 40 percent of dispensary sales in the state are attributed to concentrates. There is a loophole in the proposed law that will allow for other non-BHO methods (safer methods) to be used so as to ensure that patients who could medically benefit from cannabis concentrates still have access.

In Oregon, which currently allows medical and recreational sale and consumption of marijuana, production of concentrates without proper licensure is a felony. A government body called the Oregon Health Authority determines which dispensaries can be licensed to produce and sell concentrates.

In Washington State, where cannabis has also been legalized for both medical and recreational sale, the sale of concentrates was initially restricted. Concentrates could be sold by authorized producers to other producers who could use them to infuse cannabis edibles before selling them to the public. In other words, the average Joe cannabis consumer could not legally purchase concentrates such as BHO oil. The policy created a demand in the black market, which backfired (literally) in the form of several makeshift home laboratory explosions. A new law was passed in May of 2014 that allowed the sale of concentrates directly to consumers. The law mandated safety-related oversight over the production of cannabis concentrates. Washington's LCB (Liquor Control Board) was given the authority to conduct this oversight, and a Washington State fire marshal is now required to sign off on every new concentrate-producing facility before the onset of production.

Canada has one of the most relaxed policies toward concentrates, having legalized them fully on the basis of the patient's right to consume cannabis without having to resort to smoking, which could be damaging to the mouth, lungs, and throat. Though there are reports and complaints of prolific (and horrific) laboratory explosions in the country—especially coming out of conservative Alberta where the police force still maintains a "Team Green" devoted to busting grow-ops—it's not clear whether the law, as it stands, negatively or positively affects this public safety hazard.

Cannabis oil is a resin-like complex of cannabinoids extracted from the cannabis plant using solvents. Its final form is a solid or heavily viscous mass. The oil also bears quasi-scientific and street names, among them "hashish oil," "sativa bho," "full melt," "honey oil" or "budder." In terms of potency, cannabis oil leads the pack as the most potent of the main cannabis products because of its high THC content, which can vary depending on the plant. Various studies suggest a widely ranging THC oil content, moving between 30 percent for "homegrown" product and 99 percent for the most heavily processed.

There are several common ways of using cannabis oil, including dabbing, smoking, and eating it. The most popular is vaporizing, using an "oil rig," which is a miniature water pipe. The user heats a ceramic or similarly heat-resistant surface, puts on it a drop or bit of oil ("dabbing") and inhales the released vapor through the pipe.

Extracting resins from cannabis buds using solvents, a process not without physical danger, makes the oil. When butane is the chosen solvent, it is passed through a tube filled with cannabis plant matter. Removing the residual butane using vacuum and heat further processes the resulting mixture, called "butane hash oil." The finished product's texture determines its name: "wax," "shatter," and so forth. Solvent purity is essential for avoiding health problems.

No matter the solvent chosen for this type of extraction, fires and explosions are becoming increasingly common as more states legalize medical use of cannabis products. The danger lies in the volatility of the solvents and the failure of do-it-yourself manufacturers to follow safety procedures. Solvent fumes in the air assure instant ignition from the tiniest spark, including those generated by electric fan motors.

The now-outdated United Nations Single Convention on Narcotic Drugs, Schedules I and IV, consider cannabis oil to be a narcotic. Questions about oil's legality vary by country and within them by jurisdiction, as do fines and prison sentences. In all areas, cannabis products, oil included, are constantly moving legal, medical and social targets.

The Dawn of Dab

Perhaps the most popular method for consuming cannabis oil is "dabbing." This method of ingestion has been around for well over a decade, but the recent proliferation of cannabis concentrates has caused dabbing to surge into new heights of popularity. Dabbing involves placing cannabis oil or some other cannabis concentrate on a nail, heating it up (usually with a blowtorch), and inhaling the vapors through a glass rig.

If you're not familiar with dabbing, then it may come across as the latest "shocking new trend" that's captivated modern youth. Were you to witness it from afar, you'd see a cannabis user blowtorching an elaborate glass contraption and sucking out the resulting vapor. This same cannabis user would soon become incredibly high. Dabbing hastens the pace of cannabis intoxication to a breakneck speed.

Some in the community are concerned about the impressions left on outsiders by dabbing. Vancouver comedian Daryl Brown makes note of this in his routine, claiming that dabbing has turned weed into a "hard drug." If you've visited a dab-friendly venue then you've likely noticed a highly sedate, red-eyed opium den type of vibe—not necessarily the best impression you want to be making on a general public that's just coming around to a more enlightened attitude toward cannabis.

The popular strain-cataloging website, Leafly, notes that the advent of dabs has finally made it possible to legitimately overdose on cannabis, a phenomenon that's not good for the legalization movement. Though dab "overdoses" aren't fatal, they can result in serious injury from dabbers who pass out after consumption. Dabbing may also create particularly unpleasant highs, and there are reports of heightened after-effects and withdrawal symptoms.

Leafly goes on to discuss the upsides of the dabbing method, how patients who require high-potency medical relief have, in dabbing, an indispensable tool. Pain relief through dabbing is fast and thorough. Proponents of dabs are also quick to point out that when cannabis oil rather than cannabis flower is burned, the resulting vapor contains no plant matter and is therefore easier on the lungs. Furthermore, better vaporizers are being introduced that will eliminate the need for blowtorch ignition.

Dabbing has also permeated cannabis culture, leading to a new crop of young cannabis enthusiasts and activists, preferring the dab as their weapon of choice. Cultural events such as the Cannabis Cup have recently integrated dab-related showings and competitions into their repertoires. Meanwhile, the poor aesthetics of dabbing, coupled with the undermining of the narrative purporting cannabis to be safe and gentle, has led state legislators to take notice. In several lawmaking bodies across the country, dabbing is under the gun and could be surgically removed from the legal cannabis canon.

| 3 |
An Overview of Production

Process Overview

Cannabis or "hash" oil is an increasingly popular source of THC highs. While making it is more complicated than stuffing product into a hookah, it is not exceedingly difficult. The basic process involves a liquid solvent and cannabis leaves and buds. In the process, resins are dislodged and liquefied. The liquid is captured in a container. Since solvents are extremely volatile, they are boiled off, leaving crystalized resin, the cannabis oil. The oil is then put into a vacuum chamber to purge solvent residues. The length of this process determines the texture of the final product—in street lingo, "wax," "crumble," "shatter" and "budder."

Below are the individual steps for one of many at-home oil manufacturing methods.

Preliminaries

Distinguish between hemp and marijuana. Both plants are related, but the latter contains more cannabinoids. From it come the female buds needed for potency. Also, understand the difference between hemp oil and cannabis oil. Hemp oil is a pressing of hemp seeds, a commonplace item in health food stores; cannabis oil is a concentrated drug.

While certain cannabis oil manufacturing processes are considered relatively safe if conducted outdoors, the most popular method, using butane as a solvent, is exceedingly dangerous. Here, liquid butane is forced through a pipe filled with cannabis plant matter. As it drains down into a container it extracts the resins. Over this roughly ten-minute interval, the air immediately around the apparatus is extremely flammable.

Explosions and fires connected to butane extraction are increasing, particularly in the states where medical marijuana is legal. The early months of Colorado's legalized marijuana industry saw a quick rise in explosions and injuries resulting from attempts to manufacture the oil under unsafe conditions. Since January 1, 2014, the date of legalization, the state's burn center has treated ten seriously burned individuals who were attempting the process. Hence, public safety officials are struggling to deal with the questionable legality of the process. Legalization has complicated punishing these chemical efforts. The question is: are these individuals committing felonies, or is making cannabis oil now legal?

Law enforcement officials, in particular, have compared making the oil to running the meth labs of the '90s. Firefighters, who are often the first responders to these do-it-yourself (DIY) laboratories after the disasters, are left in a quandary as well.

Here are some examples of how cannabis oil making went wrong. Remember, in California medical cannabis products are legal.

- Close to SeaWorld San Diego in late January 2014, a hotel explosion shook the ground after an oil-making adventure failed. Guests ran for safety. Areas of the would-be oil manufacturer's skin were burned loose. Two other people were also hurt. Officials called the scene "a war zone."

- A West Hollywood cannabis-oil-related apartment explosion blew out doors and windows. Robert Bockoff, a 39-year-old DIY manufacturer, suffered third degree burns and four felony counts.

- Three men suffered burns over 80 percent of their bodies when a butane apparatus went rogue in their Los Angeles home. The explosion ignited and ultimately razed their ceiling.

- A San Francisco apartment explosion caused by cannabis oil manufacturing burned a woman and her twelve-year-old son so badly he needed face and body skin grafts.

- A January 2014 cannabis-oil-related explosion in a California apartment complex caused lengthy hospital stays for two individuals and left 140 tenants homeless.

- A Sacramento cannabis oil fire risked the lives of ten children, burned a fireman, and killed two dogs.

A California law enforcement official said, in response to episodes such as the above, "To me, it's like having somebody manufacturing bombs next door."

Medical personnel concur. Shriners Hospitals for Children's Northern California location has treated nearly seventy butane fire victims since 2011. A doctor described these accidents as "an epidemic."

Cannabis Oil Varieties

While we've already drawn a distinction earlier in this chapter between hemp oil and cannabis oil, there are, in fact, several other methods and varieties of oil production to consider. A multitude of methods and core ingredients abound, suited for various purposes.

Here are a few:

BHO

Up to now, this text has largely focused on the production and use of butane hash oil, also known as "honey oil" and "BHO." The potency and production calamities associated with BHO production keep it in the forefront of cannabis oil discussions. Creating BHO is relatively simple, albeit dangerous and, in most areas of the country, illegal. BHO is highly concentrated and can induce a profound psychoactive effect with only a moderate dose. Medically speaking, BHO is a powerful stress reliever, analgesic, and mood enhancer.

CO2 Oil

CO2 oil is currently regarded as the purest product available in the cannabis oil lineup. The reason for such acclaim is the ability of cannabinoids and terpenes to avoid degradation during the production process. The reason CO2 oil isn't as popular as BHO is that it's not as easy to make and requires specialized equipment that's not readily accessible to any would-be home chemist. The relatively low critical point of CO2 makes it an effective solvent. The critical point of a substance refers to a temperature at which its solid and gas states are indistinguishable. Once the critical point has been surpassed (along with the critical pressure), CO2 will adopt the expansion properties of a gas while retaining the density of a liquid. Compared to other solvents, extracting chemicals out of a CO2 solvent can be accomplished with very little damage. There is also considerably less adverse environmental impact with CO2.

Another interesting feature of the CO_2 extraction method is that the pressure on the solvent can be manipulated to effect different results. This more granular level of extraction control allows chemists to fully separate terpenes from cannabinoids. Compared to butane hash oil, which has an average 3 percent terpene mass, CO_2 extractions have about 10 percent.

This level of granular control allows manufacturers to craft oils for patients with very specific properties. The level of THC, for instance, can be lowered and CBD increased to accommodate a patient who does not want to experience psychoactive effects but wants a powerful pain reliever.

CBD Oil

"CBD oil" is a blanket term used to describe any cannabis oil with a high concentration of CBD. If you're purchasing CBD oil, then don't expect any noticeable THC content. Creating CBD oil can be done in a variety of ways. Using the CO_2 as the solvent is, of course, the most gentle and preferred method.

Consumers turn to CBD oil when their primary interest is medical use. CBD's properties as an anti-inflammatory, antioxidant, anticonvulsive, and anticancer agent (along with a host of other medical benefits and very limited side effects) make CBD a medical godsend.

Even states with exceptionally strict medical cannabis laws will often permit patients to access CBD oil. Contact your state's department of health to find out more.

Tinctures

fig. 4

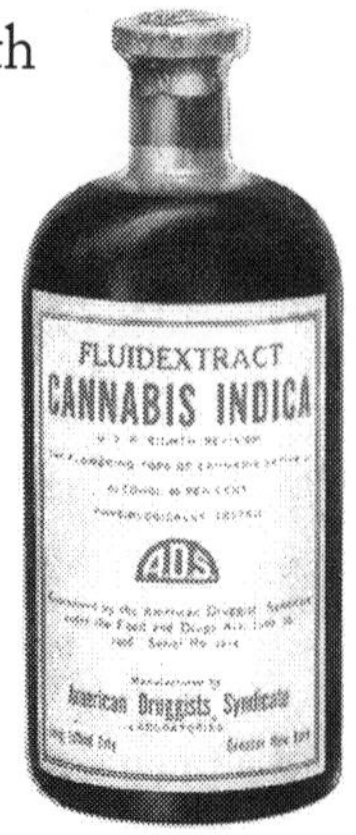

Cannabis tinctures refer to alcohol infused with cannabis. They are created by mixing alcohol together with your favorite strain of cannabis in a process similar to that used to create Rick Simpson Oil (described below). Tinctures were actually a mainstay in pharmacies in the pre-prohibition era.

Tinctures are an often overlooked but immensely valuable addition to the medical cannabis canon. They are administered by placing a few drops under the tongue via a dropper. The effects come within a few minutes, much faster than those of edibles. This short turnaround time between ingestion and effects is useful for newcomers to cannabis who are looking to find their preferred dosage level. Thus tinctures combine the best of both worlds: the ease of titrated dosage (normally associated with smoking and vaping) and a lack of irritation to the lungs and throat.

Many medical cannabis retailers specialize in tinctures, such as Tyler Strause's Randy's Club, which uses a proprietary mix of hemp oil called Cannaka™ which is specially designed to produce rich, therapeutic, and relaxing medical relief. Tyler's inspiration for Randy's Club derives from his experience caring for his father, Randy, while he was terminally ill with an incurable form of brain cancer. Along with his brother Brendon and mother Linda, Tyler sought out cannabis-derived medicines that could alleviate the symptoms of both the disease and the ensuing radiation therapy. While many of the treatments proved effective in improving Randy's quality of life, the lack of standardized products available in California's medical cannabis market was disconcerting. Randy's

Club was created with the objective of developing reliable, effective cannabis medicines, medicines that Tyler and his surviving family members "wish were available when Randy was alive."

Rick Simpson Oil/Phoenix Tears

Popularized by the modern folk legend Rick Simpson, the Johnny Appleseed of cannabis oil, Rick Simpson Oil (RSO) is made from soaking cannabis in isopropyl alcohol. RSO is truly the "open source" version of cannabis oil, as it can be made by most anyone. Here is the essential rundown of the production process (more on Rick Simpson and his medical cannabis campaign against cancer in Chapter 10):

Precautions

Be sure to conduct this operation in an area that's well ventilated—outdoors is the safest bet. Flames, sparks, and red-hot elements can pose a fire hazard, since the fumes released will be highly flammable. The fumes are also unhealthy to breathe, yet another reason for thorough ventilation or outdoor production.

Process

Ingredients needed:

- 2 buckets
- 1 ounce of dried cannabis
- A 2x2 piece of wood or something else that can be used to crush the cannabis
- 500 ml isopropyl alcohol

Place the cannabis inside one of the buckets. Use the alcohol to dampen the cannabis. Crush up the cannabis with the wood or another crushing tool. Add more solvent to the mixture until your cannabis is completely submerged. Use the wood or crushing agent to continue to crush and stir the cannabis while it's still in the solvent. Next, pour the solvent into the second bucket—just the alcohol, not the cannabis. Pour fresh oil into the original bucket to again submerge the cannabis, and continue to crush and stir the cannabis in the new mixture for another three to four minutes. Afterward, pour the solvent from the second wash into the second bucket (the same bucket containing the solvent from the first wash).

If you attempt a third wash, then you will not end up with a solvent of the same potency. As a best practice, separate your third wash solvent into a third bucket, and you can use the resulting oil for more minor medical conditions.

Simpson claims that the first wash will absorb 75 to 80 percent of the medical resins and that the second wash will absorb most remaining resins, and thus the solvent from the first wash will have the highest potency. All of which, of course, can be affected greatly by the quality level of cannabis used.

The next step is to set up a filtration process. Simpson recommends using clean water containers and a funnel, positioning the funnel at the entrance of the container and then placing a coffee filter inside the funnel before pouring the oil mixture into the funnel. The filtration process should separate all remaining plant matter from the mixture. If your remaining liquid has a coloration similar to or darker than gasoline, it's a sign that you're using good quality cannabis.

Next you'll want to boil off the solvent so you will be left with the undiluted oil. You can do this using a standard rice cooker with settings for both high and low heat. This may create fumes, so you will need to set up ventilation and fans as needed. Simpson notes that rice cookers are designed to automatically switch between low and high heat in order to avoid burning the rice. This flexibility also helps in preventing the oil from being damaged.

The key benchmark temperature to remember is 300°F (148°C). After the oil surpasses this temperature, the cannabinoids begin to vaporize and will lose their medicinal value. A rice cooker should automatically adjust its heat setting as soon as the oil reaches 210° to 230°F (100° to 110°C). Simpson discourages using slow cookers because it's difficult to regulate the level of heat that these appliances exert. In an ideal world, a distilling device would prove the most useful tool, but Simpson acknowledges that the average person doesn't possess the requisite knowledge to operate a "still" and that they're illegal to own in some parts of the country.

The fumes from the solvent will accumulate at the bottom of the rice cooker. This poses a potential hazard, because most cookers have one or two small vents near their base and if the fumes enter these vents it could cause a fire. Prevent this problem by using your fan to direct air flow at the rice cooker. If you aim the airflow at the center of the cooker it should scatter both the accumulated fumes near the bottom and the fumes that are wafting up near the top of the device. Simpson, who has completed this process "hundreds of times," says that the lowest setting on a multi-speed fan should suffice to clear out the fumes. It's important to always use a fan during this process. If enough fumes are allowed to accumulate at the base of the rice cooker, then even the heating element of the cooker itself could potentially ignite the fumes.

45

You should begin the process with the rice cooker filled approximately three-quarters to capacity (three-quarters full with the oil solvent mix). This will allow the fumes to boil off without any spillage of the liquid in the process.

As the solvent boils off, you should replenish it with your remaining oil mix, careful never to fill it past the three-fourths capacity mark. Once you've used your entire supply of solvent, allow the mixture to boil down until you have only two inches remaining. At this point, you should add ten to twelve drops of water, which will facilitate the burning-off of the last of the solvent. The water will also serve to wash away some of the solvent residue from the oil. During this final burn-off, you may notice what appears to be smoke emanating from your newly separated cannabis oil. This is not smoke, but steam that was formed by the water you added.

You will know that the solvent has been almost completely boiled off when you hear a crackling sound from the last remaining quantity of oil left in the cooker. You will also see a lot of bubbling near the end of the process.

Simpson says that after the rice cooker automatically switches to the low setting, he allows the mixture to cool off before manually toggling the cooker back to its high setting. Then, after the cooker automatically shifts down to a lower setting for the second time, he pours the contents of the inner pot into a stainless steel measuring cup.

It will be difficult or impossible to fully remove all oil residue from the rice cooker's inner pot. To clean out the pot to the fullest extent possible, use a piece of dry bread to sponge up the oil while it's warm. You can then use pieces of this bread as edible medicine. Simpson says that he personally enjoys keeping the leftover oil in the pot and saving it for future batches. In this way he combines several different strains into one oil batch so as to concoct more comprehensive healing solutions, with wider varieties of terpenes and cannabinoids.

Simpson also advises caution and temperance when consuming the oil itself or the bread used to absorb the oil left in the pot: "Even a very small amount may put you to sleep for quite a few hours." For newcomers to cannabis oil, the level of potency may indeed be astounding.

After you've poured the oil into a stainless steel cup, you should, in most situations, subject the oil to another finishing process. Simpson claims that some strains will be ready for consumption as soon as they're poured out of the cooker for the first time, but most will need to be placed on a gentle heating device, like a coffee warmer, so that the water that remains in the oil can evaporate. While on the gentle heater, the oil will bubble as the water evaporates off. Certain terpene varieties present in the cannabis strain may lengthen this boiling process. As an alternative to using the coffee warmer, you can set your oven to 250°F (120°C) and let the oil "bake" for thirty to sixty minutes.

After this secondary heating process is complete, the oil can be drawn into syringes or applicators (while still hot) then allowed to cool. The oil will thicken as it cools down, resulting in a heavier, greasy consistency that is ready to be consumed.

In our ingredient list above, we assumed one ounce of raw cannabis for 500ml of oil. This ratio can be scaled up or down as needed. For example, in Simpson's description of appropriate quantity for his recipe, he suggests eight to nine liters of solvent per pound of raw cannabis.

The entire process will take about three hours. The oil will last for a very long time, though if your intention is long-term storage, Simpson recommends using a dark bottle with a tight lid or a stainless steel container.

To reemphasize, you should be aware of the risks posed by undertaking this process and assume full responsibility for your own safety. You should also be aware of existing laws that regulate the production and consumption of cannabis oil. A survey of existing laws is available in the second chapter of this book. However, please don't rely on this book as a legal guide. Contact an attorney or your department of health. Even in the most stringently conservative states, such as Georgia, legally sanctioned provisions are available for patients seeking cannabis oil.

| 4 |

Knowing Your Growing

So, perhaps you've thought about growing your own plants for cannabis oil production. The good news for aspiring cannabis growers is that marijuana is an easy plant to grow and cultivate. It is simple to maintain and is strong enough to survive a wide range of growing conditions. This is an asset to growers who farm the plant outside of the bounds of the law, and many have become adept at growing in the most unlikely of conditions.

Cannabis is a type of plant known as an annual. Annuals complete their life cycle in a single growing season. This means that in the wild they die off for the duration of the winter and sprout anew in the spring.

For the grower this means that the annual cannabis can be planted from seed, grown to maturity, and harvested in one season. In reality, however, due to selective breeding and careful cultivation, the hardy cannabis plant can be kept alive for much longer than a single growing season and can be harvested for many years if developed properly.

Cannabis is further identified as a flowering annual, and its flowers are the plant's method of reproduction. The flowers—often referred to as buds—are also the source of the highest concentration of the psychoactive chemical, THC, and this portion of the plant is harvested for recreational or medicinal use. While there are numerous cannabinoids present in the plant's buds, THC is the most potent and is often the most sought after.

The basic needs of a cannabis plant are light, water, sufficient nutrients, and an environmental temperature kept between 70 and 80°F (21–27°C). When these needs are met, the cannabis plant can grow for many years and provide the grower with yield after yield of potent buds. Though there are a variety of strains from which a grower can choose, there are two primary types of cannabis: *Cannabis sativa* and *Cannabis indica*. The chemical properties of each of the plants are beyond the depth of this book, but we'll look at how the two varieties generally differ.

fig. 5

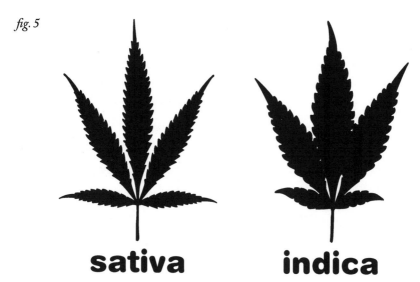

sativa   **indica**

Cannabis indica grows as a short and stout plant. Users claim that the effects of this plant are often more calming and relaxing. *Cannabis sativa* grows as a taller and narrower plant. It is often said to produce more of an energizing and stimulating effect. It is important to note that an incredible number of variables can affect the way users experience the effects of consuming marijuana. The effects vary from user to user, but some variables include personality, frame of mind, intent, experience (or naiveté), method of consumption, and tolerance.

Stages of Growth

The cannabis plant grows in three major stages: germination, vegetative growth, and flowering. From these major stages, growth can be further broken down into six more basic stages: seed, initial growth, seedling, initial vegetative growth, pre-flowering, and flowering. See fig. 6 for a summary of the growth stages along with their estimated durations.

fig. 6

Stages of Growth for the Cannabis Plant

Germination		
Seed	**Initial Growth** (1 - 21 Days)	**Seedling Stage** (7 - 21 Days)
- Seed is planted in soil	- Roots are formed - Two initial leaves	- Plant is established - New leaves are established
Vegetative Growth		
Initial Vegetative Growth (2 - 3 Months)		**Pre-Flowering Stage** (Up to 14 Days)
- The plant grows taller - The stem starts to become a stalk		- Development of calyx - Growth slows

Germination

The first basic stage of growth is called germination. In this stage the seed is in the initial stages of growth. The seed's outer layer breaks open and a root erupts from within the seed. The germinating seed continues to form roots that push downward into the soil or other growing medium. Above the soil two of the initial leaves begin forming and growing upward. We all know the basics: roots hold the plant in place and gather nutrients and water from the soil while leaves collect sunlight and perform respiration. The germination stage of a cannabis plant lasts anywhere from a day to three weeks.

Seedling

Now that the initial leaves are growing upward, they can absorb light and provide energy to the developing plant. This powers the growth of additional leaves and the development of a discernible central stem from which the leaves branch out. The seedling stage of development may last as little as one week or as long as three. During the seedling period, the plant develops four to eight leaves.

Vegetative Growth

Now that the plant is established as a seedling, it begins the stage known as vegetative growth. It continues to grow taller, and the thin stem becomes bulkier to form a stronger stalk. Not only are more leaves growing, but the leaves mature further to demonstrate the characteristic marijuana shape. Vegetative growth occurs over a period of a few months.

Pre-Flowering

The production of flowers is necessary for the plant's reproduction, but it is also highly consumptive of the plant's energy. With an expanded root system and more leaves to gather light, the plant begins to fill out and prepare for flowering. Vertical growth is reduced during this stage because the plant is directing its efforts to the production of flowers instead of reaching toward the light source.

In terms of botany (the scientific study of plants), a calyx is the plant structure that eventually becomes a bud, which identifies the sex of the plant. In the pre-flowering stage, the plant begins to show signs of its sex. In preparation for flowering calyces, it begins to grow where individual clusters of leaves meet the stalk. Calyces on cannabis plants are small protrusions that mature within the flowering stage. Pre-flowering may occur over a period of up to two weeks.

Flowering

The flowering stage is the final stage of the plant's growth cycle. This stage lasts from four to sixteen weeks and is the level at which a plant's sex is clearly visible. When the plant produces flowers, the shape of the flower determines its gender. Male plants produce clusters of small balls that become pollen sacs. Female plants produce pistils that resemble fine hairs. Pollination occurs when the male pollen sacs burst and pollen carrying the genetic material of the plant interacts with the pistils on the female buds.

fig. 7

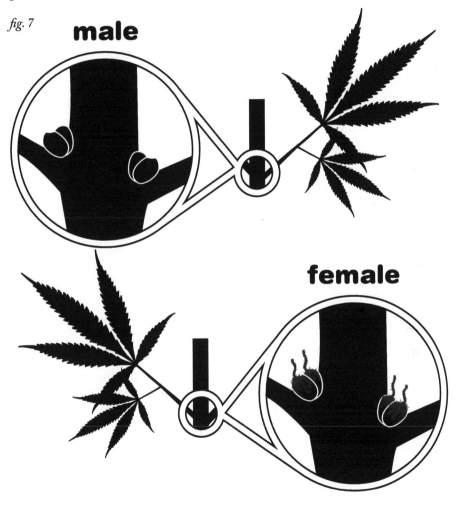

male

female

After the flowering phase of the plants, pollinated female buds produce seeds that mature within the fertilized buds for about another sixteen weeks. When the seeds reach maturity, the pods burst and the seeds drop. In the wild, the seeding process ensures that future generations of cannabis plants return the following growing season after dying off for the winter. Remember, cannabis plants are annuals.

Importance of Gender

So what if one plant is male and another is female? What does that have to do with anything? The answer is *everything*. It is extremely important to understand how to sex your plants to ensure the most productive crop yields.

We already know that cannabis plants are annuals, but they are also dioecious, meaning that plants produce either male or female flowers but not usually both. The opposite of dioecious is monoecious, meaning a plant that has both male and female flowers present on the same plant. There are rare instances of cannabis plants that are hermaphrodites, with male and female organs present in each bud or both sexes of flower present on a single plant.

While it may sound advantageous to have cannabis plants that will self-pollinate or a room full of both sexes that will propagate much faster, the opposite is more desirable for growers, especially for-profit growers. If the plants are being cultivated for recreational or medicinal purposes, then the concentration of THC present in the buds will be the chief indicator of quality. When male and female plants are mixed within a generation, or even within an entire crop, it can have a profound and negative effect on the levels of THC that are found within the harvested buds.

The pollination or reproduction process of the cannabis plant involves male pollen sacs bursting and the pollen transferring genetic material to the pistils of the female bud. Once the female bud is fertilized, it begins to produce a seed. The problem with this scenario is that once a female plant is pollinated, it directs all of its energy to the development of the seed. Once the seed is growing, the levels of THC produced in the bud drop off and the result is a much less potent product. When the female plant is deprived of male pollen, the female develops ever stickier, more potent buds so as to give her the best possible chance of capturing any available male pollen. Oddly enough, what's known to marijuana growers as a potent, high-value plant is in fact an example of botanical female sexual frustration.

As a grower, you want to cultivate a high-quality, potent product no matter what its end use will be. A quality product can command a higher price, and the process of separating your male and female plants is relatively easy.

Sexing Your Plants

A farmer who raises livestock will tell you that if you want to know the sex of one of your sheep, just lift the tail. Not so easy with plants that have neither tails nor what we would recognize as genitals.

If you are starting a crop with a random batch of seeds, it is likely that you will have an approximate split of 50/50 male and female plants. There is no way to tell which sex the plant will be as a seed; the first indicators only come once the plant reaches the pre-flowering stage. It's easiest to identify the gender of a plant once it has completed the flowering stage, but by then it may be too late. The males may have successfully pollinated the female plants, and an entire crop, or at least a portion of it, may be ruined.

Remember calyces? They'll begin to form in the fourth or fifth week of growth. (To refresh your memory on the entire growth cycle, refer back to fig. 6.) Close inspection of these soon-to-be buds is key to successfully separating your plants early enough to avoid accidental pollination. This is critical to the successful growth of marijuana, and thus this is neither the first nor the last time the visual indicators will be mentioned.

fig. 8

Gender Differentiation Signs

male	female
Calyx will produce signs of pollen sacs	Calyx will produce signs of pistils
Pollen sacs resemble small balls	Pistils resemble fine hairs

You may not want to wait until your plants reach the flowering stage before identifying their sex. Cultivating an entire crop of plants requires time, effort, and resources. It's not prudent business to spend time and money growing a crop of plants only to discard half of them. This could effectively double the cost of growing your plants before you could correctly sex them, so identify the gender as soon as possible to save time and money.

The following are quick sex identification techniques. Keep each of these in mind when sexing your plants, as they are not all guaranteed to be 100 percent accurate—where one may not work, another could save you time and money by weeding out males quickly and leaving the THC-rich females unfertilized. The exception to this rule is cloning, which is a little more involved and highly reliable.

Rate of Maturation

A basic indicator can be the time it takes each plant to show the signs of its sex, otherwise known as maturing. Females will often take longer to show signs of budding, so if a bunch are showing signs of being male and the others are taking their time, this in itself can be an indicator of which plants are female.

Buying All-Female (Feminized) Seeds

What if you could avoid growing males in the first place? Growing from a batch of female-only seeds will ensure that you spend less time worrying about the gender of your plants. Methods of producing all-female crops for seed sale are outside the scope of this book, but some sellers may be able to provide presorted seed batches for larger growing operations. Be aware: even in a female-only batch of seeds, a male or two, or several, may still pop up, so pay attention.

Size

Another early sexing technique is observing the size of your plants as they grow. Male plants tend to be larger than the female plants that were planted at the same time and have grown under the same conditions. While this is generally considered to be quite effective for distinguishing sex, it is not 100 percent guaranteed that female plants will be smaller, so keep that in mind.

Cloning

Cloning plants is the only true way to guarantee their sex. A clone will have the exact same DNA as its host or parent, and therefore the exact same sex. While this is the most involved and time-consuming method of sexing your cannabis plants, it is also highly accurate and the only reliable way to ensure correct gender identification.

The cloning process involves taking a small cutting of the parent plant. The cutting is placed in soil and allowed to grow on its own for a few days before it is forced into early flowering through a process of being exposed to twelve hours of darkness and twelve hours of light. This is done apart from the host plants; they should be allowed to grow normally without forced flowering. Once the clones begin to flower, their sex—which will always correspond to that of their parents—can be verified.

Sprout Location During Germination

While this is perhaps the least scientific of all the early sexing methods, many growers claim that they can identify the sex of their plants with 90 percent accuracy just by observing where the sprout emerged from the seed. It is the experience of many growers that top or bottom sprouts result in female plants, whereas side sprouts result in male plants. Don't start throwing away all your side-sprouting plants just yet; keep a log of your plants that sprout sideways and see if they end up being males. If you are seeing consistent numbers, consider using this method of early sexing. Some growers trust it to the extent that all side-sprouting seeds get discarded immediately, while others are more suspicious of the consistency of the results.

Hermaphrodites

Keep an eye out for plants that exhibit both pollen sacs and pistils. If these occur, try pruning off the male calyces in an effort to train the plant to develop only female flowers. A hermaphroditic plant could potentially self-pollinate or pollinate other nearby plants due to the presence of the male flower and its pollen sacs.

Growers who are producing marijuana for recreational or medicinal purposes will be harvesting from the female plants, the ones that produce the highest levels of THC. The earlier males can be detected, the lower the chances they have of pollinating the females and the fewer resources are consumed raising useless plants. Once the males are separated they can be destroyed, or they can be reserved to pollinate more females in the interest of breeding your next crop.

Try different methods and evaluate the results for yourself. Cloning is the most reliable method, but it takes time and resources. We all know that time is money, and money is money, so if you can determine a method that's quicker and gives you a level of reliability with which you're comfortable, that's the best choice for you.

| 5 |
Legal Considerations

Whether you grow your own plants or purchase what you need to make cannabis oil, it's important to know that each country has its own rules related to cannabis products; even within countries there may be differing laws for each region. In general, possession of the oil is forbidden. However, across the globe, the oil and other related products' medicinal powers have created confusing situations and a puzzled citizenry. What's legal now? What isn't?

Currently, many individuals, organizations, etc., throughout the world want to legalize cannabis products. They are certain this will stamp out drug dealing, provide new sources of tax revenue, and cut enforcement costs. Already, Canada has approved these products for medicinal use. Public resistance to legalization in the United States has dropped. The most recent national polls indicate that 56 percent of voters are pro-legalization.

So it was not a total surprise when, on November 6, 2012, Colorado and Washington State passed laws to legalize recreational use of cannabis. Alaska and the District of Columbia followed suit in 2014, fully legalizing the possession of small amounts of marijuana by adults. Yet the federal government still classifies it as a Schedule I controlled substance, which means punishment for those who possess it. When Governor John Hickenlooper of Colorado officially signed the bill into law, he felt he was part of a great historical event. He said, "Certainly, this industry will create jobs. Whether it's good for the brand of our state is still up in the air. But the voters passed Amendment 64 by a clear majority. That's why we're going to implement it as effectively as we possibly can." Further studies in Colorado suggested a $60 million state benefit from combined savings and taxes.

On the international scene, Uruguay became the first country to attempt to include cannabis in its above-ground economy, the effort beginning in December 2013. The head of its National Drug Council specified government production control. Vetted companies would be permitted to vie for cultivation licenses. To further tarnish free marketers' optimism, the government would control all aspects of the operation. Purchase of a maximum 40 grams would be allowed for those eighteen or older, once registered. Limits on production would exist as well: a maximum of six crops annually, total production limited to 480 grams. Smoking clubs would have the privilege of growing ninety-nine plants. No foreign purchases were allowed. No cross-border drug movement, either. However, President Jose Mujica delayed implementation until 2015, citing "practical difficulties" with this government-grown cannabis proposition. Today, home growers/sellers are still an issue and there aren't enough law enforcement officials to deal with the problem.

Many countries in the world are far from adopting the Uruguayan attitude. For some of them, dealing in drugs, including cannabis oil, means death to the offender. For example, in Saudi Arabia, a hashish smuggler was executed in 2005. Indonesia launched a very real war on drugs when it instituted the death penalty for drug doings in 1997. Curiously, no major drug dealers have met justice, despite former President Megawati Sukarnoputri having threatened, "For those who distribute drugs, life sentences and other prison sentences are no longer sufficient. No sentence is sufficient other than the death sentence."

Malaysia executed two men in 1996 for selling a little more than one kilogram of cannabis. In 2004, a Japanese person who smuggled more than 1500 grams through Philippine airport security was sentenced to life in prison. In Brunei, a Malaysian was hanged for being found with 992 grams of cannabis. Having 600 grams or less would have spared him. Thailand, Singapore, and China have no compunction whatever about the death penalty when it comes to drug trafficking. More enthusiasm for executions is exercised in the People's Republic on or near the United Nations' International Day Against Drug Abuse and Illicit Drug Trafficking.

Washington State, Alaska, Oregon, the District of Columbia, and Colorado have legalized cannabis products for recreational use. However, a late-2012 poll showed that 64 percent of responders felt the federal government should take no action at all in regard to the use of recreational cannabis. As expected, the younger the polled individual, the more they favored legalization.

Internationally, reform means loosening restrictions through treaties. The most recent UN Single Convention on Narcotic Drugs placed cannabis firmly in the deepest circle of condemnation, Schedule IV. Nonetheless, changes in the categories of drugs can be made through tedious procedures. The legalization of recreational cannabis in the United States provoked a United Nations complaint. The International Narcotics Control Board (INCB) urged Washington to challenge the legalizations. INCB President Raymond Yans called them violations of the Single Convention. The US Attorney General responded in December 2012 that growing, selling, or possessing any amount of marijuana remained illegal under federal law. President Yans described the response as "good but insufficient." He hoped Congress would work to comply with existing drug control treaties.

Of course, cannabis oil regulations and penalties vary across the world. Australia's Northern Territory fines individuals $200 for possessing up to one gram of oil. Payment inside of twenty-eight days cleans the slate. In New Zealand, any cannabis-processed substance is considered a Class B drug. Italian law only issues a warning for possession of up to one gram of THC; subsequent infractions are dealt with more harshly. Portugal disallows drug processing apparatus and consumption tools. It does allow individual possession of 2.5 grams or less of cannabis oil. In the United Kingdom, hashish is a Class B controlled substance, but oil is now entangled in the law over issues of nomenclature: "liquid cannabis" or "hash oil," "purified form" or "solvent extract," and so forth.

In summary, US laws against cannabis oil and other products are largely rigid, though states have taken initiatives for which the final implications may not be resolved until years in the future. It is virtually certain that the worldwide use of cannabis oil for medical purposes is in the cards. Already, cannabinoid derivatives such as dronabinol and nabilone are commercially available. CBD oil, a THC-lite compound, has been approved for use in ten states. However, those hoping for recreational use of cannabis oil across the continent may have a long wait.

| 6 |

General Immediate Effects

As a direct derivative of cannabis, the oil has the same chemical characteristics as its source, but in greater concentration. Like cannabis, the oil contains cannabinoids, in particular tetrahydrocannabinol (THC). Large doses of THC can produce hallucinations and affect the human body in other ways. While many fear that cannabis use produces negative effects, such as schizophrenia and depression, among other issues, various studies have produced only ambiguous results. Federal regulations further limit medical use investigations. Similar scientific forays into damage to long-term memory have been confounding.

As mentioned, THC is the key psychoactive in all cannabis products. Industrious selection and nurture can produce yields containing up to as much as 29 percent of this cannabinoid. As well, cannabis contains related compounds that, in themselves, are not psychoactive, but seem to be required for THC to operate in the human body. They are thought to affect metabolism by reducing body temperature and influencing immunity and cell protection. Natural cannabis oil holds terpenoids or "terpenes" (discussed in Chapter 1) that may combine with cannabinoids to produce the anticipated results. In the body, THC quickly becomes 11-hydroxy-THC, allowing the effects to continue even after blood level THC has dropped. While not generally known as a cannabis benefit, it seems a better antioxidant than either vitamin E or C.

In the brain the cannabinoid receptor is one of the most common, identified as "G protein-coupled," and greatly abundant. In Chapter 1 of this book we discussed the body's naturally occurring endocannabinoid system and how cannabinoid receptors and neurotransmitters were discovered in the early 1990s. Scientists soon discovered that cannabinoids found in cannabis (phytocannabinoids) had the same effect on the brain as chemicals that exist naturally in the body (endocannabinoids). These cannabinoid receptors now appear to be commonplace, not just throughout the human body, but in most other vertebrates and invertebrates as well. In fact, recent evidence suggests that their evolutionary path winds back 500 million years. Cannabinoids are assumed to play a part in the brain's control of motion and recall, as well as reducing pain. They attach to the body's fatty tissue, thereby extending the time the compounds are held in the body, up to ten days for the occasional user.

The near-seamless integration of phytocannabinoids into the living tissue of an organism, coupled with the impossibly high threshold for cannabis-based toxicity (overdose), makes cannabis far less risky than alcohol and a multitude of pharmaceutical drugs. The idea of cannabis as a threat to life is completely unsubstantiated. A 2001 review in the *British Journal of Psychiatry* claimed that "no deaths directly due to acute cannabis use have ever been reported." The plant's toxicity is quite limited. Administering lethal doses to laboratory animals is virtually impossible. As to humans, a fatal dose of cannabis is 40,000 times as much as one that is needed to reach a maximum high.

Cannabis and tobacco smoke have been compared on a toxicity basis. While similar, cannabis smoke is more heavily laden with ammonia, hydrogen cyanide, and nitrous oxides compared to that of tobacco, though recent studies contradict these findings, suggesting a lesser disparity. In any case, cancer-causing agents like lead, arsenic, and polonium-210 are largely absent from cannabis smoke. Despite this, there are enough residual tars to tag cannabis smoke as carcinogenic, according to a 2012 California government report. However, it falls well below tobacco smoke as a cancer-causing agent. Its use, even when relatively frequent, does not compare with the product consumption of an addicted tobacco smoker.

When vaporized and inhaled, cannabis oil's effects begin at once. They are fully felt in a minute or two. The high lasts from one to three hours, based, of course, on the individual's constitution and the potency of the oil. Oral consumption via cannabis-infused food or drink delays impact in exchange for a longer high. Repeated use almost guarantees cannabinoid tolerance.

When discussing the nature of a high, subjectivity and method reign. Technically, this is what happens. THC passes from the lungs into the bloodstream. In the brain it hooks up with many receptors. The changes in the receptors alter neurotransmitters, chief among them dopamine and norepinephrine, causing users to experience anxiety, euphoria, or various combinations of the two. Additional effects reported are altered perception, joyfulness, calm, giddiness and musical discernment. Many experience episodic memory, rising sensuality and libido, and the urge to philosophize. For nearly a third of users the downside is anxiety, often accompanied by panic attacks. Frequently, the senses are heightened: food tastes better, music sounds sweeter, and comedy is funnier. Time perception grows uncertain. Some users indulge heavily in search of a dissociated or depersonalized state, even at the cost of later panic attacks and paranoia. Mental disturbances diminish after five to seven hours. Heavy users can be afflicted for days. Extreme cases require restraint and sedation. While cannabis serves as both a stimulant and a depressant, its predominant properties center on generating hallucinations and psychedelic activity.

Cannabis oil users may also experience rising pulse rates, dry mouth, bloodshot eyes and hot or cold extremities. Motor activity is reduced. When oil is taken orally, the high takes longer to develop, but lasts as long as ten hours. Of course, oral ingestion avoids danger to the lungs.

Cannabinoids find their way to the basal ganglia and the cerebellum where motor skills are supported and controlled, and to the hippocampus, which is the seat of learning and memory. In addition, the cerebral cortex, the region of sophisticated thinking, is affected, as is the nucleus accumbens, the brain's gratification center. To a lesser degree, cannabinoids affect the hypothalamus (homeostatic functions), the amygdala (emotions and fears), the brain stem (sleep, arousal) and the nucleus of the solitary tract (digestive disturbances). Evidence indicates cannabis use disturbs short-term memory by reducing the production of neurotransmitters in the hippocampus, resulting in reduced neuronal activity.

fig. 9

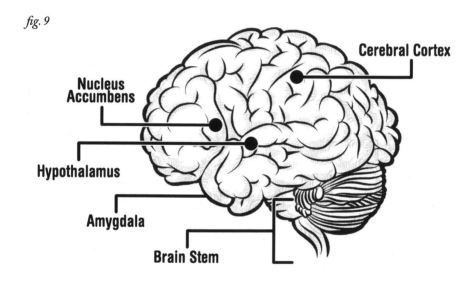

It is not safe to drive after cannabis use. The *British Medical Journal* reported that those who indulged up to three hours before taking the wheel were twice as likely to cause an accident as a sober driver. The United Kingdom's Department for Transport identified young male drug and alcohol users as a traffic accident risk group. Their driving inexperience, attitudes toward taking risks, and attitudes in general may be connected to both using drugs and accident risk, thus skewing the drug-use accident-involvement statistics. Nonetheless, a cannabis-using driver is an impaired one.

The European Monitoring Centre for Drugs and Drug Addiction observed in 2008 that "even in those who learn to compensate for a drug's impairing effects, substantial impairment in performance can still be observed under conditions of general task performance." Impairment, however, is relative. In 2013 a group of sixty-eight separate drug-related crash risk studies was analyzed to measure the impact of various drugs—cannabis, cocaine, amphetamines, and so forth. Researchers concluded, "By and large, the increase in the risk of accident involvement associated with the use of drugs must be regarded as modest . . . Compared to the huge increase in accident risk associated with alcohol, as well as the high accident rate among young drivers, the increases in risk associated with the use of drugs are surprisingly small." Supporting this study was another study from three western US universities revealing that the legalization of medical cannabis reduced traffic fatalities by nearly 11 percent. The reason is that drunk drivers are more reckless; cannabis users understand their driving skills are compromised, so they drive more carefully.

In terms of heart health and cannabis products, younger users need not fear. It is older users who are taking some risks. The *International Journal of Cardiology* reported in 2007 that cannabis use generated a host of myocardial infarction triggers, such as increasing heart workload and postural hypotension. A study from Boston Beth Israel Deaconess Medical Center, Massachusetts General Hospital, and Harvard School of Public Health found that a middle-aged person's heart attack risk climbs almost five times in the first hour after cannabis use. Research into such use is hampered by the presence of other drugs, specifically alcohol and nicotine, and, as was mentioned in Chapter 1, "elevated heart attack risk" can be tied to several normal healthy activities such as sex and exercise. The lack of improved controls leaves open the possibility that that certain symptoms of cannabis use might in fact be attributable to tobacco, particularly when pressures provided by the funding source, say a pro-tobacco institution, invite weird science. Many say raw data alone should be the target for examination. Understandably, the proponents of cannabis legalization maintain persistent vigilance in the face of seemingly damning reports touting cannabis-related harm. This is of course due to the decades-long history of propaganda and misinformation that's fueled the failed prohibitionist policy.

Studies on the effects of cannabis products have targeted short-term memory. In a 2001 study, researchers found that while some cognitive gaps were visible seven days following use, they were reversible. After twenty-eight days, memory shortcomings disappeared. In their 2003 investigations, University of California, San Diego (UCSD) School of Medicine researchers could not show meaningful systemic neurological effects from long-term cannabis usage.

Studies headed by Dr. Igor Grant, a UCSD professor of psychiatry and director of the Center for Medicinal Cannabis Research, looked at the safety and efficacy of using medicinal cannabis to treat diseases. The team found that the drug did affect perception, but it did not cause irreversible brain damage. Researchers analyzed fifteen earlier studies featuring more than 700 long-term cannabis users and nearly 500 non-users. The results revealed that long-term use was only slightly harmful to memory and learning, and there was no effect on other cognitive functions like reaction time and motor skills.

Harvard professor Harrison Pope said his researchers found marijuana not to be dangerous in the long-term, but not without short-term effects. Pope's tests disclosed that long-term cannabis users had a hard time with verbal memory in particular for "at least a week or two" after ingesting the cannabis product. After a month, memories were back to normal.

Matters of appetite are commonplace in cannabis users' experiences. The abrupt urge to eat has been investigated in both the United Kingdom and the United States and found to be real and the result of hypothalamic action. As such, cannabis medicine has been put to use as an appetite stimulant on behalf of cancer patients and those suffering from other appetite-suppressing disorders.

Compared to more common methods of cannabis consumption, cannabis oil has a reputation for being highly potent. Newcomers are shocked to find that even a small amount of oil can have profound effects, especially when the cannabis strain used to create the oil is high in THC. Persons who overconsume may experience an unwanted severity of psychoactive effect, including anxiety, paranoia, and even hallucinations. If you're uncertain as to what effects to expect from a certain strain or are uncertain as to an appropriate dosage, then you'll fare better using a cannabis oil tincture as opposed to using baked goods or candies as a delivery mechanism. While it may take thirty minutes to an hour before you notice any effect from cannabis-oil-infused edibles, the fast-acting tincture will begin to act within minutes, and you can adjust your dose accordingly.

| 7 |
Long-Term Effects

Because cannabis oil and related cannabis products are largely illegal, research on their benefits and detriments has been considerably limited. Nonetheless, a body of information exists on which one can rely, at least for the present.

Excessive consumption of cannabis products is a risk to the memory and intelligence of children and young adolescents. Long-term adult use, barring great overdosing, poses no such problems. Nevertheless, there is a modest risk of psychological dependence that spans all age groups. Itai Danovitch and his colleagues in their 2012 article in *Psychiatric Clinics of North America* pointed out that only 1.8 percent of users can be medically defined as dependent. Of all who first begin to use cannabis, only 9 percent are ever likely to grow dependent. While no known medicine can relieve dependency, psychotherapy and motivational modification are sometimes successful. Addiction potential is lower than that of cocaine and heroin, but higher than for hallucinatory drugs like LSD.

While cannabis products do not directly cause mental illness, they may play a role if the subject is already susceptible. Understandably, early and frequent use opens the door to later psychological problems. Researchers contend that THC's permanent damaging effects are muted by CBD. As with mental illness, cannabis products themselves do not cause acute psychosis, but can figure in the illness of someone already predisposed. Such dispositions might include genetic tendencies or previous mental or physical trauma. Schizophrenics' thinking processes have been improved after cannabis use, but no evidence exists that it either improves or worsens the schizophrenic condition. Considering cannabis as a catalyst for depression seems valid only under conditions in which individuals begin use early in life and continue for years. Similarly, incidence of suicide is more likely in the group of early and long-term users; otherwise, suicide rates are comparable with those of non-users.

The graphic below lists several other hazards associated with long-term cannabis use.

fig. 10

Potential Harms Associated with Long-Term Cannabis Use

Reduced resistance to common illnesses	Suppression of the immune system
Growth disorders	Increase of abnormally structured cells
Reduction of male sex hormone	Personality and mood changes
Apathy/lack of motivation	Inability to understand things clearly

Suggestion that cannabis products' use causes academic underperformance in secondary schools is subject to question. Yes, studies by the National Household Survey on Drug Abuse and Arrestee Drug Abuse Monitoring program data suggest weaker academic performance and high dropout rates among users, but this information is unreliable. At the college level, grades and achievements were the same for users and non-users, though the former were more indecisive about a career path. Possibly surprising is 2011 and 2013 evidence presented in the *American Journal of Epidemiology* that cannabis users are less likely to be obese, have healthier insulin systems, and have better "good" cholesterol measurements.

Getting Ahead of the Gateway Theory

The idea of cannabis products as "gateways" to harder drugs has been prevalent for decades. However, supporting evidence for this supposition has been elusive. "Dueling" studies are commonplace. Some suggest that the real gateway drug is alcohol; others note that many hard drug users have used neither cannabis nor alcohol. No less an authority than the National Academy of Sciences reported, "There is no evidence that marijuana serves as a stepping stone on the basis of its particular drug effect." Not long ago the Canadian Senate Special Committee on Illegal Drugs declared, "Cannabis itself is not a cause of other drug use. In this sense, we reject the gateway theory."

In light of these findings about the gateway theory, along with its tendency to be associated with antiquated advocacies of the "DARE" movement, the gateway theory does get a bad rap, perhaps unfairly so. To summarily dismiss the much-maligned gateway theory could be intellectually disingenuous at best, and at worst, harmful. The antagonist bias toward the gateway theory has in large part been a knee-jerk reactionary response to the antagonistic bias against cannabis itself. Couple that with the painstaking difficulties involved in moving beyond correlation to show causation when it comes to gateway drugs.

Detractors of the gateway theory are apt to argue that the criminalization of cannabis results in a greater likelihood of cannabis users coming into contact with street dealers who also traffic in cocaine, ecstasy, and other drugs "beyond the gateway." What's missing at the moment is data that shows definitely that cannabis consumers who purchase through legal channels are more likely than non-cannabis users to use other drugs. But dismissing the gateway theory wholesale is premature and even unlikely. Attempting such a dismissal becomes incredibly complicated when confronted with drug culture at-large, the literature, media, and communities such as MAPS, VICE, *High Times* magazine, Ibogaine clinics, shamanist churches of ayahuasca, and countless others that embrace a very open-minded view of a multitude of mind-altering substances, cannabis et al. These cultural associations and co-exposures will surely persist past the point of legalization, making it quite naïve to assert that one's choice to engage in the experience of cannabis has zero bearing on one's choice to engage in the experiences offered with other mind-altering drugs. To make such an assertion, in a certain sense, would be to disavow much of what makes cannabis such a potent cultural symbol: the idealism, peace, healing, righteous rebellion, and mind expansion believed by cannabis consumers to be inherent to the experience itself. Those who exist in the thick of cannabis culture would never allow their drug of choice to be relegated to the status of an effective but otherwise boring medicine, legal or not. Since ancient times, cannabis has held meaning, for some, of a profound and spiritual nature. Consumption of cannabis surely does affect one's willingness and curiosity regarding experimenting with other drugs. Rather than summarily dismissing the gateway theory, we should work to extract the concept from the jaws of the politically-charged drug war and seek instead an objective view. And objectively speaking, 60 percent of people who consume cannabis will go on to consume other drugs; 43 percent will go on to consume drugs other than alcohol.

A multitude of compelling theories abound concerning the relationship between cannabis products and hard drugs—some of which are based on the cultural associations described above, while others have their roots in the failed propaganda campaigns of the drug war. Regardless of the source, the existence of gateway drug usage should be acknowledged for what it is, and attempts to ignore the facts on the ground so as to protect the reputation of cannabis should be curtailed.

Here are some common gateway theory arguments that link cannabis to other drug use:

1. Some suggest that there are individuals who look to get high on anything and find cannabis products among the easiest to find. Many high schoolers, for instance, find it much easier to obtain cannabis than to obtain alcohol, even in states with stricter laws.

2. The young see warnings against cannabis product use as exaggerated, so they dismiss anti-drug warnings. Serious, life-threatening drug addiction, believe it or not, was one of the major casualties of the drug war. When people began to discover that they'd been lied to about cannabis's dangers, risks, and lack of value, they grew to distrust and reject wholesale the tidings of the drug war. This in turn led to a lack of seriousness and good judgment when it came to using other, more dangerous drugs.

3. Social groups of gateway drug users overlap those using hard drugs. That's just the way it is, and it could very well continue even in a society that's more legally and socially tolerant toward cannabis use.

Alcohol as a Gateway

You can't have an objective discussion about gateway theory without mentioning alcohol. Alcohol use commonly precedes indulgence in other drugs, including cannabis products. Drinkers are much more likely to use drugs, at the following rates: cocaine, 26 percent; cannabis, 14 percent; psychedelics, 13 percent. Drinkers take to drugs at a rate six times greater than that of nondrinkers.

Other Gateway-Related Items of Note

Perhaps the gateway drug issue with the heaviest objective health toll is that which is associated with tobacco consumption. More than 60 percent of drug abusers smoke tobacco, which is three times the rate of the general population. This data makes way for the argument that a person's heightened risk of smoking tobacco could very well be the most dangerous side-effect of smoking pot. And which one is illegal again?

| 8 |

Medicinal Treatment : An Overview

Putting aside today's jurisdictional and legal confusions regarding the use of cannabis oil and other cannabis products as medicine, history from ancient times forward confirms their potency. Present day use centers largely on reducing nausea and vomiting, as well as pain reduction. The establishment is uncertain about related adverse effects, long-term use, thinking and memory gaps, and child safety. The oil is either eaten or vaporized and inhaled. Anecdotal use includes direct application to afflicted areas. Synthetics like dronabinol and nabilone are in use in North America and Europe. In the United States, nearly two dozen states allow medical use, though the federal government still upholds its Controlled Substance Act (part of the Comprehensive Drug Abuse Prevention and Control Act of 1970), maintaining that any use is illegal.

The Upside

Indeed, cannabinoids in whatever form can improve appetite, reduce vomiting and nausea, curb spasms, reduce pain, and ameliorate AIDS symptoms. Nonetheless, both the Food and Drug Administration (FDA) and the National Institute on Drug Abuse dismissed marijuana itself as an "unlikely medication." A 1999 study of cannabis health benefits nixed smoking as a treatment, but allowed that the substance was useful in reducing nausea, improving appetite, and reducing pain and anxiety. Researchers found fault with existing delivery mechanisms and the shortage of clinical research data, so much so that the American Society of Addiction Medicine declared in 2011 that cannabis medical applications should be ended, even in states where legalized.

Chemotherapy-induced nausea and vomiting (CINV) in adults and children can be reduced with cannabis when preferential treatments fail, despite the side effects of a high. Claims of successful treatment of AIDS/HIV remain unsubstantiated for reasons of limited samples, bias, and inadequate long-term data.

Pain reduction superior to that of opiates appears to be one of the less controversial areas of cannabis product effectiveness. Neuropathy, fibromyalgia, and arthritis sufferers have all found relief through medical cannabis products, though side effects remain an issue. The situation is much the same concerning cannabinoid use in the treatment for multiple sclerosis, epilepsy, and motor difficulties. THC combined with CBD reduces spasticity. Ten countries allow cannabis treatment for multiple sclerosis.

fig. 11

Suggested Medical Applications for Cannabis

AIDS	Anxiety
Arthritis	Cancer
Chron's Disease	Epilepsy/Seizures
Fibromyalgia	Glaucoma
Irritable Bowel Syndrome	Ménière's Disease
Multiple Sclerosis	Nausea
Parkinson's	PTSD
Rheumatism	Sleep Disorders

The Downside

Cannabis product enthusiasts tend to overlook the many adverse effects, among them a negative impact on mental, social, and physical health. Use also has been connected to liver disease and lung, heart, and vascular problems. There is agreement that cannabinoids have medical value, but such value is prone to becoming maligned in the eyes of the general public when the drug is flippantly prescribed and the lines between medicine and recreation become blurred. The FDA and others in the scientific community would like to see the same rigorous testing of cannabis as is done on newly developed drugs, a process sometimes requiring fifteen years.

According to the National Institute of Health's (NIH) current findings, cannabis has an adverse effect on concentration. Users experience a reduced ability to perform tasks that require coordination and have a generally more apathetic attitude toward personal productivity.

Perhaps Comedy Central's *South Park* put it best:

> *"The truth is, marijuana probably isn't gonna make you kill people, and it most likely isn't gonna fund terrorism, but... pot makes you feel fine with being bored, and it's when you're bored that you should be learning some new skill or discovering some new science or being creative. If you smoke pot you may grow up to find out that you aren't good at anything."*

Another piece of age-old wisdom that comes into play when taking stock of the downsides of cannabis use is "what goes up, must come down." The NIH finds that cannabis users may feel depressed when coming down from their high and that irritability and anxiety ensue. It's certainly not the crippling and violent kind of withdrawal that addicts experience with heroin, but nonetheless, these negative effects are documented facts.

There are countless cannabis users who, though they may not meet the technical criteria for addiction, rely on the heavy, daily consumption of cannabis for their basic day-to-day functionality. Many of these heavy and frequent consumers do not have any substantive medical condition to speak of, other than a dependence on (if not an addiction to) cannabis.

Cannabis & Youth

There has been much talk in recent years about the effects of cannabis on neurodevelopment in adolescents and young adults. Before we get into the hard numbers, let's first consider the predicament of the adolescent cannabis user. The late teenage years and early twenties are often associated with the formation of key components of self-identity. At this age we're confronted with the prospect of leaving home, of pursuing a trade or higher education, and of thinking seriously about the future. The cannabis experience provides (for most) a kind of relief from the mundanities and obligations that life imposes on us. And the method used with cannabis is one of deconstruction, a viewing of one's life through an altered lens. Fundamental beliefs and personal values are all called into question and, as French poet Charles Baudelaire puts it, "The relation between ideas becomes so vague, and the thread of your thoughts grows so tenuous, that only your cohorts... can understand you." Baudelaire would eventually discontinue his own use of hashish, claiming its "annihilation of the will" in his reasoning. Again, consider the plight of adolescents: their development of fundamental beliefs and values, and their modality for expression of the will, are all approaching critical depths during these formative years. From a narrative-psychological perspective, it's apparent how possible it is that cannabis could aggressively disrupt the functioning and growth of a young mind.

Now, let's look at the data. A Northwestern University School of Medicine study found that cannabis use by young adults created abnormalities in two regions of the brain that support emotion and motivation. The study also found that the extent to which these abnormalities were present directly correlated with the frequency of cannabis use. It was also found that those who began using cannabis after the age of twenty-one did not usually experience these adverse effects. The American Psychological Association (APA) reports that similar findings abound on the impact of cannabis use on the brains of young adults.

In addition to scientific study, we must also take into consideration associative data—that which shows a *correlation* between cannabis use and other factors but is not sufficient to suggest a direct *cause*.

The APA also found that a host of "poor life outcomes" were associated with heavy cannabis use at a young age:

- Higher dropout rates
- More likely to depend on welfare
- More likely to be unemployed
- Less overall satisfaction with life

Politically speaking, the subject of cannabis still suffers from a vast divide of ignorance between those who judge its value (or lack thereof) by its negative associations (many of which are surely the product of criminalization) and those who've grown to so distrust society's institutions that they remain willfully ignorant of any and all proposed harms associated with cannabis.

As is the case with so many facets of the great cannabis debate, what we need most are objectivity and an openness to facts and common-sense solutions.

| 9 |

Use for Diseases & Disorders

While there have been claims of cures attributed to the use of cannabis in a variety of forms, the truth is that even some of the most staunch supporters of cannabis use for medical purposes claim only that the substance helps address various symptoms of a variety of diseases.

These claims have been valid enough to prompt twenty-three states and the District of Columbia (at the time of this printing) to allow the use of medical cannabis. Possession limits vary from state to state and are expressed as the amount of "usable" cannabis one is allowed to have, how many plants an individual can possess, or sometimes by the amount used daily, for example a sixty-day supply.

Other states, not on that list of twenty-four, have passed legalization laws that permit physicians to "prescribe" marijuana, and additional states have passed what are known as "affirmative defense" laws, which allow arrested marijuana users to offer medical use as part of their defense.

Nonetheless, no matter how one acquires cannabis, there is indeed historical and documented evidence of its successful interaction with a number of diseases. Below is a profile of each of those diseases/disorders and how the substance is used in the context of treating it.

DISCLAIMER: The authors of this book are not medical doctors and do not specifically recommend cannabis for the treatment of any of the diseases or disorders listed below. This dissertation is merely a compilation of the ailments for which treatment with cannabis has proven to be effective for relief of symptoms. This book does not claim that cannabis oil or any other cannabis derivatives will cure the ailments listed herein. Anyone considering the use of cannabis as a treatment for a particular disease should consult with their doctor/specialist or an expert in the use of cannabis for medicinal purposes.

Diseases & Disorders

Alzheimer's Disease

In the United States alone, an estimated five million individuals have been diagnosed with Alzheimer's disease, a (usually) age-related disease with which many are all too familiar. It causes serious cognitive decline, robs the victim of their memories, and often affects that victim's behavior, prompting agitation and sometimes violent outbursts.

Experts note that some aspects of the disease might be interwoven with an individual's endocannabinoid system, indicating that, eventually, some successful treatments for Alzheimer's could be cannabinoid-based. It is hypothesized that THC could potentially slow the buildup of plaques in the nervous system.

Currently, however, cannabis taken orally is recommended to calm agitated Alzheimer's patients and to stimulate their appetite and help them sleep. A recommended amount is five to ten milligrams; higher amounts could actually cause agitation. *Vaporization* is suitable as well, but only under direct supervision. Recommended plants are the Purple and Afghan broad-leaf varieties, because they are high in THC.

Anxiety Disorders

This is a tricky one, though many anxiety sufferers will tell you that cannabis oil has helped them immensely. The caveat is that large doses of cannabis can prompt anxiety, paranoia, and other such episodes, no doubt causing setbacks for those who had hoped for relief. But those who tout its use for anything from panic disorder to OCD to PTSD say that if care is taken to choose the correct variety (strain) of plant and the right dosage, then the likelihood of relieving the symptoms of anxiety is quite high.

Smoking and vaping are the chosen methods for addressing anxiety with medical cannabis. It is recommended that the patient start with a dose only as large as a match head in order to avoid sedation. They must completely vaporize the active ingredients of that micro-dose. Bubba Kush is the recommended type for general anxiety, while CBD varieties are excellent for social anxiety, phobias, and panic disorder.

Arthritis

The historical record shows that cannabis was used to treat arthritis as long ago as about 2500 BC, when it was included in the recommendations of ancient Chinese pharmacists. There's also evidence from first-century England that it was used to restore "the softness of joints." This is possible thanks to the fact that CBD works as an anti-inflammatory, which is exactly what the arthritis patient requires. Hence, it's used to treat pain.

Oral cannabis for arthritis treatment is an excellent choice because its effects are long-lasting, but smoked and vaporized cannabis have also been used with success. Researchers are also looking into the possibility of a topical form of cannabinoids and whether or not that would be even more effective. Consider high-THC and high-CBG varieties for daytime pain relief that won't put the patient to sleep. Blending those with a high-CBD cannabis can provide even more anti-inflammatory effects.

Autism Spectrum Disorders

Autism (and other disorders that fall into the same category, such as Asperger's) is classified as a pervasive developmental disorder that impairs social interaction and communication. Children said to be on the "autism spectrum" have differing abilities to interact with others, and many exhibit aggressive and agitated behavior, sometimes to the point of violence.

Use of cannabis to control these anxious and aggressive behaviors is quite controversial, but many doctors are advocates for its use or, at the very least, advocates for further research into the use of cannabis to treat children on the autism spectrum. Others merely support the rights of often-overwhelmed parents to try experimenting with cannabis as a treatment for autism spectrum symptoms.

A professional must recommend dosage for each particular child based on factors such as the child's reaction to other drugs, his/her age, and specific factors of the child's disorder (for example, what kinds of symptoms appear on a regular basis). Vaporized cannabis has shown the most success but, of course, must be done under close parental and medical supervision. High myrcene and linalool varieties are recommended due to their anti-anxiety properties.

Cancer

For specific information on cannabis and cancer treatment, refer to Chapter 10.

Chronic Fatigue Syndrome

Chronic fatigue syndrome is a mystery to many, including much of the medical world. It is characterized—as the name indicates—by very severe fatigue accompanied by joint pain, impaired memory and concentration, sore throat, headache, and sleep that leaves the victim unrefreshed and seemingly ushers them into yet another day of misery. Its cause has been attributed to everything from viruses to toxins.

Though no formal studies have been made regarding the effectiveness of cannabis to treat chronic fatigue, some believe that chronic fatigue is a result of oxidative stress, which causes damage to cellular components. Reports show that CBD-rich cannabis can reduce the symptoms of oxidative stress. Hence, cannabis flowers rich in CBD are recommended for vaporization.

Diabetes

A 2013 issue of the *American Journal of Medicine* included an editorial that contemplated whether or not THC would one day be commonly prescribed for individuals with diabetes and other metabolic disorders. It was prompted by the fact that a recent study had indicated healthier levels of insulin in cannabis users as compared to nonusers of cannabis. Due to the rising number of diagnoses of diabetes in the United States and the number of individuals who are said to be pre-diabetic, these findings were deemed ultra-important, especially by those who promote medical cannabis use.

Though the ability of cannabis to address the underlying causes of diabetes is still being researched, promising results such as those mentioned above have prompted many to give it a try. It is hypothesized that diabetic complications that are linked to the endocannabinoid system can be lessened with the use of cannabis. These include blindness, kidney failure, heart disease, and neuropathic pain. Plant cannabinoids with no psychoactivity may also assist in maintaining pancreatic function and insulin resistance.

Dosage will vary depending on the variety of cannabis used, and further research will assist in targeting the most effective varieties of cannabis for the treatment of diabetes. For now, studies show that varieties high in CBD and another cannabinoid called tetrahydrocannabivarin (THCV), when vaporized, may be the best bet.

Fibromyalgia

Similar to arthritis, fibromyalgia is a rheumatic disorder that causes chronic pain. Symptoms are generally attributed to problems with the nervous and endocrine systems, social or environmental stressors, or genetics. Cannabis may be used to treat not the underlying cause of the disorder but, rather, its symptoms.

Dosage should be controlled so that psychoactivity is not prompted. According to reports, the experience of most patients is that four milligrams of THC is effective. Look for varieties of cannabis classified as THC or CBD chemotypes.

Gerontology

Obviously, being old isn't a disease or a disorder, but aging comes with many medical issues that can be addressed through the use of cannabis. Common uses among the senior population are for treatment of insomnia, arthritis, depression, appetite issues, and, as previously indicated, dementia-related diseases. A variety of studies show that cannabis use among the over-sixty crowd is bigger than ever, basically because that population is the same population that used marijuana as a recreational drug in the 1960s.

Older adults need to realize, however, that how their body reacted to cannabis forty or fifty years ago may not be how it reacts today. For that reason, proper dosing is essential and it's always preferable to underdose. Vaporization is a good way to control the dose, and it also allows for quick results. Look for relaxing varieties rather than stimulating ones for most senior-related problems.

Glaucoma

The use of cannabis to treat glaucoma was lauded back in the 1970s when a study discovered that smoking marijuana lowered intraocular pressure. It is that pressure that builds up and damages the eyes in glaucoma, because the fluid within the eye, as a result, does not move as it should. This eventually causes blindness. Those who are critical of cannabis use for glaucoma say that the effects don't last long enough; that is, the pressure is only relieved for a few hours at a time. The same group of skeptics argues that regular users also build up a tolerance to THC and that it stops working.

Nonetheless, there is some evidence that small doses will be effective, at least for a short amount of time, helping to stay the eventual result of glaucoma, which is blindness. High-CBD varieties are suggested and can be administered orally, smoked, or vaporized.

HIV/AIDS

There's plenty of history between cannabis use and AIDS/HIV. That's largely because the early years of the medical marijuana movement and the early years of the AIDS epidemic coincided.

According to Michael Backes, who penned *Cannabis Pharmacy: The Practical Guide to Medical Marijuana,* cannabis was immediately tapped to help stimulate the appetites of AIDS patients and prompt weight gain, and to reduce their nausea, usually caused not only by the disease but by the medications they were given. Volunteers would distribute edible cannabis products (brownies, etc.) to AIDS patients in the most affected places, like San Francisco General Hospital.

Today, HIV patients can live long and fairly healthy lives, thanks to the approved medications that have hit the market in the last fifteen to twenty years. No longer is HIV a sure death sentence. However, cannabis can still be used to address neuropathic pain associated with the disease as well as drug-related nausea and loss of appetite. Ultra-high-THC varieties work well for nausea and appetite stimulation, and high-CBD varieties are good for neuropathy.

Insomnia

Because a lot of cannabis-based medicines can cause sedation, they have been used often to treat insomnia and sleep apnea. In addition, because many sleep disorders are caused by pain-related disorders, they react well to the anti-inflammatory properties of cannabis.

However, some cannabis types promote wakefulness instead of sedation, so varieties and dosages must be chosen carefully so as not to trigger the opposite effect in insomniacs. In the instances where cannabis does prompt sleepiness, it sometimes takes sixty to ninety minutes for that to happen, so those who wish to vaporize, for example, high-THC cannabis, should do so at least an hour before they wish to sleep. But they should avoid another dose if they wake up in the middle of the night and can't fall back to sleep, because overmedicating could occur and psychoactivity might begin.

Migraines

Those who've studied migraines and cannabis use theorize that migraines are indicative of an endocannabinoid deficiency. Hence, cannabis can be employed to reduce symptoms. However, some regular migraine sufferers have used it as a prophylactic—to reduce the frequency of migraines through prevention. Reducing symptoms and preventing migraines altogether each demand different varieties of cannabis oil and different dosages. Prophylactic therapy involves taking doses during the time of day when headaches most often occur, such as mid-afternoon or in the morning. Symptomatic relief is best realized if the cannabis is vaporized or smoked in the early stages of the migraine, but definitely not before it's evident that a migraine is coming. Using it during the "aura" stage seems to be most productive, and regular users say it can keep the migraine from progressing.

Multiple Sclerosis

Where multiple sclerosis (MS) and other movement disorders are concerned, cannabis is most often used to treat the symptom known as "spasticity," an involuntary limb function that results from the fact that an MS (or other) patient does not have control over certain voluntary movements. This is caused by damaged motor nerves, which is common with not only MS but also amyotrophic lateral sclerosis (ALS) and cerebral palsy, and in individuals with spinal cord injuries.

A 2011 study at the University of London, Blizard Institute, demonstrated that cannabis can provide symptomatic relief for those suffering from spasticity by regulating the aforementioned dysfunctional nerve transmissions.

Yet another study was done recently at the University of California Center for Medicinal Cannabis Research and it was determined that, in this placebo-controlled trial, results showed a reduction in both spasticity and pain. (Many were taking other FDA-approved meds as well, including interferon.) Nonetheless, the study has been gauged as significant to the MS community, though some who have tried medicating with cannabis report only subtle differences.

Sublingual usage (under the tongue) and smoking seemed to provide the best results in treating spasticity and MS-related pain.

Nausea & Vomiting

Cannabis has been explored in the treatment of nausea and vomiting, particularly for chemotherapy patients, since the 1970s. A 1975 study in the *New England Journal of Medicine* pronounced THC as effective in reducing vomiting during chemotherapy when used by patients taking seven different standard (at the time) chemo drugs.

Today, it seems that oncologists regularly recommend cannabis for those undergoing both chemotherapy and radiation treatments. Through the early years of the new millennium, more than two dozen studies were done on the subject, and it was discovered that non-psychoactive, acidic forms of THC (found in raw cannabis flowers) may be most effective in treating nausea and vomiting connected with cancer treatments.

Specifically, cannabinoids are quite effective at reducing the sensation of nausea and also at minimizing delayed nausea and vomiting, which is commonly associated with the platinum agents used in the treatment of many different kinds of cancer. Results can be achieved through oral or sublingual doses or by smoking or vaporizing varieties such as OG Kush or Bubba Kush.

Parkinson's Disease

Parkinson's is a progressive neurodegenerative disease that is most recognizable by the classic tremors that appear in most patients. These and other symptoms are the result of decreased stimulation of the brain's motor cortex. Some of the drugs recommended for Parkinson's disease carry a huge risk of developing other movement-related symptoms, such as tardive dyskinesia, characterized by uncontrolled movements of the face, head, arms, and legs.

There is currently no conclusive evidence that cannabis can aid in the treatment of Parkinson's, but proponents of its use say that observational studies appear promising. An Israeli study conducted in 2013 showed a 30 percent improvement in patients using cannabis to control tremors, rigidity, and slowness of movement. Pain improved as well.

Smoked and sublingual cannabis have been the preferred method of delivery in most of the Parkinson's-related studies.

Seizure Disorders

Researchers have long been curious about the effects of cannabis on seizures, especially since nearly one-third of those who suffer epileptic seizures have been unaided by the anti-seizure drugs that are currently available on the market. However, studies are still in their early stages, and though the results are promising, small clinical trials continue and patients await further report.

Most of the research these days centers on the use of CBD and THCV varieties, which have few adverse side effects and no psychoactivity. Animal studies using synthetic cannabis that targets the CB1 receptor have also been successful.

Because seizure disorders and the patients they affect are so different, and because some cannabis can increase seizure activity, consultation with a physician is paramount.

| 10 |
Cannabis Oil for Cancer Treatment

The drug-conscious world is awash with anecdotal evidence of cannabis oil's efficacy as a cancer cure. Leading the list of proselytizers early in the effort was Rick Simpson, who morphed from a Canadian hospital boiler room worker to an on-the-run guru praising the oil's homeopathic potential. Experiences, first with family members and then with his own personal health problems, led him to try marijuana against his doctor's advice. Soon he was making his own cannabis oil against his own government's advice (and law). He used the oil to successfully treat a multitude of illnesses, beginning with his own skin cancer and continuing with his mother's psoriasis. He moved on to acquaintances' skin cancers, and then took on cases of glaucoma, arthritis, and high blood pressure.

According to his claims, his oil coaxed Stage 4 cancer patients away from the edge of death. Diabetic ulcers? No problem. Diabetes sufferers tossed away their insulin in favor of his oil. With the help of the Royal Canadian Legion, he carried his message and his oil to the country's veterans—at no charge to anyone. Nonetheless, the Royal Canadian Mounted Police raided his premises in 2003. Not deterred, he videotaped interviews with the many people he claimed to cure.

A typical example of such testimonials is directly quoted from *PhoenixTears.ca*, the website that touts "Rick Simpson Oil":

> *"Hey dude, scan results today, 50% or more reduction in the main mass (which was unexpected by the docs), nothing on the liver (small spot before), nothing in the brain (small spot before) nothing in the other*

lung (15 small quarter size spots before), nothing on the ribs, (c6 and c9 encased in cancer before), nothing around the heart... the doctor is freaked."

Simpson's video brought the Mounties to his door again, this time with an arrest warrant. Tried in 2007, and not permitted to introduce forty-eight sworn affidavits witnessing to his oil's successes, Simpson was found guilty and sentenced to two years in jail. He has now left Canada and continues his cannabis oil crusade elsewhere, through public speeches and seminars. He is reported to have cured 5,000 people with cannabis oil, all at no charge.

An often-repeated Simpson "case study" is that of Dusty Banks, who was diagnosed with prostate cancer in 2013. His doctor offered the usual surgery and radiation treatments. Banks then watched the previously-mentioned video featuring the story of Rick Simpson, produced by Christian Laurettes and titled *Run from the Cure*, by now a pro-cannabis-oil cancer treatment classic. Banks also checked out the related popular Internet sites, Phoenixtears.ca and CureYourOwnCancer.org. He opted for the oil cure, though he was warned against it by his doctor. He ingested a small dab three times a day for four days, after which he felt generally better. In three months, his cancer was gone. Furthermore, he claims his blood pressure lowered, a toe joint inflamed for ten years calmed, rectal bleeding and pain stopped, long-standing shoulder and spinal pain dwindled, nasal drip dried, and his need for antidepressant medicines and painkillers ended. These days, he needs only a single vitamin pill and a monthly one-gram oil "maintenance dose."

Indeed, pro-cannabis-oil sites include the results of "scientific research" into what appear to be successes in human cancer treatment. Yet, with few exceptions, the medical establishment is opposed to its use.

What, in fact, are the realities of cannabis product effects on human cancers? Not surprisingly, the American Cancer Society is not so enthusiastic about miracle-like cancer reversals. Its site warns, "Relying on marijuana alone as treatment while avoiding or delaying conventional medical care for cancer may have serious health consequences." The society's position is cautious. It suggests more cannabinoid research is necessary along with research directed at improving therapies related to tackling the side effects of cancer treatment. It speaks out against the government's insistence on maintaining cannabis as a Schedule I drug, thus interfering with research and study.

For precise information on the subject, one turns to the National Cancer Institute (NCI). While it is generally accepted that cannabinoids are useful in reducing cancer-related pain, their effects on human cancers themselves are unproven, the NCI maintains. Nonetheless, one National Toxicology Program study found that cannabinoids seemed to protect against tumor development in mice and rats.7 Over the course of two years the animals were given varying dosages of THC. The result was a reduction in liver cancer. Benign tumor counts dropped in other organs. A related study showed that THC and cannabidiol (CBD) limited the growth of lung carcinoma.

Cannabis users who have or did have cancer concur with some of these findings, of course. Others merely use cannabis to treat many of the common symptoms of various kinds of cancer and to address the side effects of often-unpleasant cancer treatments like chemotherapy and radiation. Cannabis use to treat side effects of some of the more cutting-edge treatments, like immunotherapy or gene therapy, has not been researched as of yet.

Within the context of oncology (cancer treatment) cannabis can play an important role on several fronts:

Nausea/Vomiting

Chemotherapy is the major cause of nausea and vomiting among cancer patients. While some of the newer chemo drugs aren't as likely to cause distress, some of the drugs—including the often-used varieties of so-called platinum agents such as cisplatin—are relentless when it comes to nausea. Cannabis is extremely effective as an antiemetic (anti-nausea drug) and has been used as such for several decades. Only one FDA-approved medication, Emend, comes close to offering the relief provided by cannabis.

Stimulation of Appetite

Everyone knows that marijuana gives one the so-called "munchies." Using cannabis for nausea and vomiting also allows for stimulation of appetite, something that other antiemetics don't do. As a matter of fact, it was for this purpose that the FDA approved the first cannabis-based medication, Marinol. However, Marinol prompted lots of psychoactivity, so users eventually switched to herbal cannabis options instead, which allowed them to better control the dosage.

Anxiety

Using cannabis for anxiety relief is tricky; the user will need to be sure that the dosage is high enough to reduce anxiety but low enough not to cause other psychoactivity that may be counterproductive. CBD has been the most successful for anxiety reduction, usually in doses no bigger than 5 ml.

Pain

Chemo patients suffer from debilitating amounts of neuropathic pain, and cannabis medicines can be quite useful for reducing this. A study completed way back in 1975 by Noyes et al determined that 10 mg of THC could be as effective as 60 mg of codeine over seven hours of treatment. (See more information about cannabis and pain in Chapter 7.)

Mood Elevation

THC interferes with memory creation and, as such, it seems to assist with improvement in mood, even for those with a grim prognosis or those going through difficult patches due to debilitating treatments for their cancer. There are no specific studies on this issue. Rather, "researchers" such as the aforementioned Rick Simpson have made careful note of positive mood changes in their clients.

Tumor Reduction/Antitumor Activity

Most oncologists, even those who encourage the use of cannabis for their patients, find it necessary to admit that there is no "real" proof that cannabis can cure cancer, no scientific studies that have deemed cannabis oil a miracle potion. The only thing that comes close is a 2012 Italian study using non-THC cannabinoids to treat prostate cancer. Interesting to note, individuals suffering from prostate cancer are known to possess under-functioning endocannabinoid systems. This study and others haveprompted an ongoing call for further research. However, research at the time of this writing, generalized research into cannabis as an antitumor agent hasn't been adequately pursued.

Therefore, since no *verified* scientific studies exist in which cannabinoids have been used to successfully treat human cancers, the jury of public opinion must remain unsettled and anecdotal cures suspect. Even so, cancer victims need not choose between total relying on traditional medicine's sometimes-successful cures and rolling the cannabis oil dice alone in hope of an unlikely miracle. Combining radiology and chemotherapy with cannabis treatment works for many patients, particularly in addressing disease symptoms and treatment side effects together, but a cure should not be anticipated.

| 11 |

Consumer Purchase of Cannabis Oil

Considering the dangers of manufacturing cannabis oil at home, many of its medical and recreational users turn to purchasing it elsewhere. In earlier years this required an often-illicit connection with a local dealer. Since the advent of the Internet, the situation has changed. Yes, one can buy cannabis oil and the herb itself online. A quick check on the Net turns up many "medical dispensaries," such as Harborside Health Center, Medicineman's Online Dispensary, and Cannabits. However, buying this way invites trouble. To simply sign on through a normal browser, say Google Chrome, for the purpose of buying drugs is to invite the scrutiny of the law and the possibility of being scammed, built-in "security" notwithstanding. So, buyers must understand two things. The first is that they must buy on the black market. The second is that they need to use encryption and nontraditional currency to avoid the authorities' attention.

Black markets on the Internet have existed for some time. The FBI closed two of the largest, Atlantis and Silk Road, in 2013. Silk Road 2.0 is already in business, as are unknown numbers of other decentralized black markets across the globe. To buy successfully in this relatively challenging environment requires a unique browser, such as Tor. Tor masks the user's Internet Protocol (IP) address and records no activity. Downloading and activating Tor takes less than a minute.

The alternative currency problem is solved with the use of bitcoin, a decentralized, anonymous digital currency. The most significant element of the bitcoin system is a public bitcoin transaction ledger. This is handled without central authority intermediation, as long as "mining," the method by which bitcoins are earned, is decentralized. Instead, a host of intermediaries exist as computer servers running bitcoin software. These Internet-connected devices make up a network that anyone can join. Transactions can take the form of Payer A sending N bitcoins to Payee B. Each transaction is sent to this network using commonplace software. Bitcoin servers check these transactions, add them to their copy of the ledger, and then distribute these ledger additions to other servers. Buyers must first choose a bitcoin "wallet," then buy bitcoins through a website like Coinbase. With bitcoins in virtual hand, the buyer signs on to the chosen black market site. Creating an account requires the establishment of a passphrase and PIN. Prior to any transactions, the account must be funded with bitcoin. Once done, the buyer proceeds as though signed in to any online store. In the black market store, cannabis oil and other cannabis products, including bagged marijuana, are available. It is important to remember, however, that any such transactions are completely illegal in federal eyes.

State Laws

At the time of this writing four states, Washington, Oregon, Colorado, and Alaska, along with the District of Columbia, allow the possession of cannabis for both medical and recreational purposes. Several other states have laws governing medical use of marijuana, and several more have "CBD-only" laws, allowing only marijuana products with low THC.

The map graphically summarizes current cannabis law in the United States (as of 2016), with the darker states being more liberal towards cannabis and the lighter states being more prohibitive:

fig. 12

Map of US State Cannabis Laws

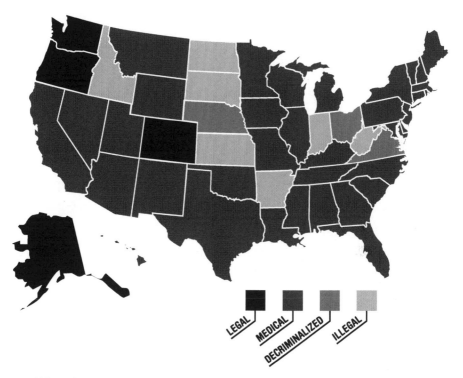

If you're looking to purchase cannabis oil through a legal channel, then you will want to familiarize yourself with the law in your state. Below you'll find a brief summary of current cannabis policy in several states:

California

Though California is in many ways synonymous with cannabis culture, as of this writing, it's been outdone on the legal front by both of its northern neighbors, Oregon and Washington. Nonetheless, California was the first state to enact a law legalizing medical use of cannabis.

Current law in California allows patients and their primary caregivers to grow and use cannabis for qualified medical use.

Dispensaries abound and it's not difficult to acquire cannabis oil or other forms of marijuana legally in this state with a medical prescription. At one point it was said that there were more dispensaries in the Los Angeles area than there were Starbucks, a noteworthy accomplishment indeed.

Texas

Texas is one of several states to permit the sale and consumption of low-THC cannabis. The program is known as the Compassionate Use Program, and though it's in effect as of January 10, 2016, it may take up to a year before a reliable infrastructure is in place to service patients.

New York

New York allows medical use of cannabis. Citizens qualify for use if they have one of a handful of diagnosed medical conditions. They are then asked to register with the state's Department of Health and afterwards they're issued a "Medical Marijuana Card."

Mississippi

In July of 2014, Mississippi passed into law a measure to allow the possession of cannabis for seizure disorders. The law stipulates that the cannabis must contain no more than 0.5 percent THC and at least 15 percent CBD. The law permits only three major research centers, and its detractors say that it's not wide-sweeping enough to really be effective. The law's proponents say that it's an important symbolic gesture by the state.

Michigan

Marijuana laws in Michigan are governed by the "Michigan Medical Marihuana Act." *(Michigan uses the old-school, prohibition-era spelling of the word: "Marihuana.")*

Patients who have a qualifying medical condition are allowed to cultivate and possess cannabis for medical use. Physicians treating a qualifying patient are also allowed to cultivate and deliver cannabis on behalf of their patients. Patients are required to register with the Michigan Department of Community Health. Once registered, they receive a registry identification card.

The Michigan law limits the amount of cannabis that a registered patient may possess to 2.5 usable ounces. The patient may keep up to twelve marijuana plants in a secure location.

Georgia

The Georgia state law governing medical cannabis use went into effect in September of 2015. The law strictly defines less than ten qualifying medical conditions and, similar to Mississippi, puts a strict cap on the concentration of THC in your cannabis product. Applicants along with their physicians are required to submit some brief paperwork to the Georgia Department of Public Health.

A successive legal measure that would allow for limited cultivation of cannabis in Georgia by state-licensed producers failed to clear the legislature. For now, Georgia patients must source their cannabis outside of the state, though the state does supply a listing of vendors who offer products that meet the THC/CBD thresholds stipulated in the Georgia statute.

Other States

Most other states that permit the medical use of cannabis have some variation of the legality statuses described above. For a thorough rundown on the applicable laws in your state, we encourage you to check out NORML.org.

conclusion

So, how will future generations view cannabis and its use? It's tough to predict. Indeed, there have been indications that the federal government is moving toward normalization of cannabis. Legalization is increasingly being thought of as a social justice issue. However, the Obama administration has gone on record more than once concerning its hands-off position as to how states want to deal with cannabis. Advocates are increasingly attacking the ranking of cannabis products as Schedule I substances, equivalents of heroin and cocaine.

Meanwhile, pro and con skirmishing will continue to fester around the usual topics: negative and positive cannabis impacts on the mind and body, cannabis vs. alcohol, and therapeutic value of the substance. The reality is that none of these issues can be finally resolved until the federal government ban is lifted and the scientific and medical establishments can conduct the necessary research and experimentation. Judging by the history behind various states' legalization, no legislative action is likely on a top-down basis. That is, Congress or the appropriate agencies will not act until nationwide sentiment forces their hand.

However, cannabis acceptance is certainly moving forward. A 2015 Gallup poll showed that 51 percent of its participants were in favor of sweeping marijuana legalization. Within the next few years, it is anticipated that Nevada, California, Vermont, Arizona, and possibly Connecticut, Michigan, and Rhode Island will legalize recreational cannabis use. Good voter turnout in the looming 2016 election could make a difference in many states, because many cannabis-related proposals will appear on the ballot in November.

The Golden State of California is among those facing a referendum on recreational cannabis legalization. "For California, you're looking at a $15 billion market potentially, and probably 15 percent of that will go back to the state coffers," said Norton Arbelaez, the founder of Denver-based RiverRock Cannabis, a chain of marijuana dispensaries. He noted that passage of the recreational marijuana law in Colorado resulted in a new industry that provided ten thousand jobs in that state. In California, he added, the impact would be enormous, merely because of the vast size of the state's economy.

Many believe (and many fear) that in the newly legalized world the cannabis industry will be taken over by "big tobacco," spelling the end of the black markets. The absence of cannabis as an illegal target could free government resources to tackle the truly harmful drugs, like heroin and cocaine. The United States could become a cannabis mecca, drawing appreciative users and their money from across the globe and doing wonders for the overall economy.

Still, others don't see that ever happening, at least not in the near future. Those watching the 2016 presidential candidates closely note that many have taken a rather apathetic approach to the question of amending the Controlled Substances Act and legalizing cannabis on the federal level, choosing a wait-and-see attitude rather than a commitment to one direction or another. Others, mostly Republicans, have expressed their opposition loudly and clearly. Meanwhile, President Obama's former attorney general, Eric Holder, has stated that the Justice Department does not intend to interfere with the state laws now in effect in Washington, Colorado, and Oregon. When Hillary Clinton was asked about her opinions on cannabis, whether she was for or against it, her response was to call for more research into the medical value and dangers of cannabis.

The recent expansion of legalization across the country, even in very limited forms such as that enacted by the Georgia legislature, does give the impression that government authority is tagging along behind the expressed will of the public. After Sanjay Gupta's groundbreaking documentary on the efficacy of cannabis as a treatment for children with epilepsy, it figures that no lawmaker wants to get in between a suffering child and her medicine. We can only hope to witness a steady convergence of science and policy, one that liberates patients and caregivers while still encouraging a healthy society.

glossary

Boggs Act-
Passed in 1952, this act set mandatory sentences for drug convictions. A first offense conviction for marijuana possession carried a fine of up to $20,000 and two to ten years' imprisonment.

CBD (Cannabidiol)-
One of many active cannabinoids in cannabis, CBD can assist in treatment of several diseases and their symptoms/side effects but does not contain the psychoactive properties of THC and other cannabinoids. Hence, the user does not feel "stoned" when using it.

Controlled Substances Act (1970)-
A federal US drug policy under which the manufacture, importation, possession, use, and distribution of certain narcotics, stimulants, depressants, hallucinogens, anabolic steroids, and other chemicals are regulated.

Hashish-
The flowering tops and leaves of Indian hemp smoked, chewed, or drunk as a narcotic and/or intoxicant.

Hemp-
Also known as Indian hemp, this tall, coarse plant is native to Asia but is grown around the world and used as a source of fiber (to make rope, etc.). It is also used to make drugs, including marijuana and hashish.

Marinol-
The first synthetic FDA-approved cannabinoid-class drug, still used to treat nausea and vomiting in chemotherapy patients and to manage appetite loss in AIDS patients.

Medical Marijuana-
Refers to the use of cannabis or marijuana, including components of cannabis, THC and other cannabinoids, as a physician-recommended form of medicine or herbal therapy.

Terpenes-
Fragrant and medically useful unsaturated hydrocarbon molecules found within a plant's essential oils.

THC (tetrahydrocannabinol)-
The primary intoxicant in marijuana. THC is a compound obtained from the cannabis plant. It produces a high level of psychoactivity in users.

Vaporization-
A technique for avoiding irritating respiratory toxins in marijuana smoke by heating cannabis to a temperature where the psychoactive ingredients evaporate without causing combustion.

references

Crawford, Vivienne, "A Homelie Herbe: Medicinal Cannabis in Early England," *Journal of Cannabis Therapeutics* 2 (2002): 71–79.

Albert, Joseph S., "Marijuana for Diabetic Control," *American Journal of Medicine* 126, no. 7 (2013): 557–558.

Baker, David, et al., "The Biology that Underpins the Therapeutic Potential of Cannabis-Based Medicines for the Control of Spasticity in Multiple Sclerosis," *Multiple Sclerosis and Related Disorders* 1 (2012): 64–75.

Corey-Bloom, J., et al., "Smoked Cannabis for Spasticity in Multiple Sclerosis: A Randomized, Placebo-Controlled Trial," *Canadian Medical Association Journal* 184, no. 10 (2012): 1143–1150.

Sallan, Stephen E., et al., "Antiemetic Effect of Delta-9 Tetrahydrocannabinol in Patients Receiving Cancer Chemotherapy," *New England Journal of Medicine* 293, no. 16 (1975): 795–797.

Lotan, I., et al., "Medical Marijuana Treatment for Motor and Non-Motor Symptoms in Parkinson Disease: An Open-Label Observational Study," *Clin Neuropharmacol.* 2014 Mar-Apr;37(2): 41-44 doi: 10.1097/WNF.0000000000000016.

Williams, Sean. "Here's Why Marijuana Probably Won't Be Legalized by the Federal Government Before 2020," *The Motley Fool.* The Motley Fool. N.p., 11 July 2015.

about clydebank

We are a multi-media publishing company that provides reliable, high-quality, and easily accessible information to a global customer base. Developed out of the need for beginner-friendly content that can be accessed across multiple platforms, we deliver unbiased, up-to-date, information through our multiple product offerings.

Through our strategic partnerships with some of the world's largest retailers, we are able to simplify the learning process for customers around the world, providing our readers with an authoritative source of information for the subjects that matter to them. Our end-user focused philosophy puts the satisfaction of our customers at the forefront of our mission. We are committed to creating multi-media products that allow our customers to learn what they want, when they want, and how they want.

ClydeBank Alternative is a division of the multimedia-publishing firm ClydeBank Media. ClydeBank Media's goal is to provide affordable, accessible information to a global market through different forms of media such as eBooks, paperback books and audio books. Company divisions are based on subject matter, each consisting of a dedicated team of researchers, writers, editors and designers.

For more information, please visit us at :
www.clydebankmedia.com
or contact info@clydebankmedia.com

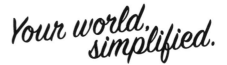

notes

STAY INFORMED

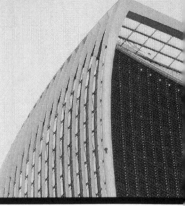

ClydeBank BUSINESS | BLOG

Your Source for All Things Business

Why Should I Sign Up for the Mailing List?

- Get a $10 ClydeBank Media gift card!
- Be the first to know about new products
- Receive exclusive promotions & discounts

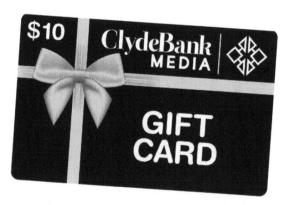

Stay on top of the latest business trends by joining our free mailing list today at:

www.clydebankmedia.com/business-blog

DOWNLOAD A FREE AUDIOBOOK

Get a **FREE** ClydeBank Media Audiobook + 30 Day Free Trial to Audible.com

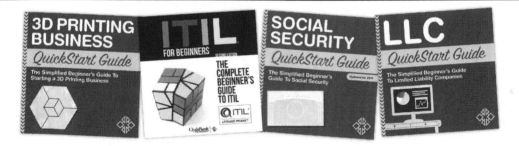

Get titles like this absolutely free :

- Business Plan QuickStart Guide
- Options Trading QuickStart Guide
- ITIL For Beginners
- Scrum QuickStart Guide
- JavaScript QuickStart Guide
- 3D Printing QuickStart Guide

- LLC QuickStart Guide
- Lean Six Sigma QuickStart Guide
- Project Management QuickStart Guide
- Social Security QuickStart Guide
- Medicare QuickStart Guide
- And Much More!

To sign up & get your FREE audiobook, visit:

www.clydebankmedia.com/free-audiobook

81515187R00071

Made in the USA
Middletown, DE
25 July 2018